KETO Diet Cookbook for women over 50

Only truly Keto Low Carb recipes to be Wonder Woman

(carbs max 5 grams, with pictures!)

By Michael Bone

1. Introduction

In many ketogenic diet books, people complain that many recipes were written just to fill the pages, but that they are not really keto recipes. I have personally seen recipes that had 30 grams of carbohydrates for each serving.

In this Keto Diet Cookbook for women over 50 you will find only truly Keto recipes. We are talking about recipes with a carbohydrate content of less than 5 grams, which will help you change your metabolism, lose weight in a short time, and feel fitter.

On the following pages you will find answers to some of the most frequently asked questions about keto diet.

That's it ... turn on your cook mode and enjoy!

2. Celebs who love the Keto Diet

Halle berry, 54 years old actress hasn't been shy about her love for the keto diet. She told *People* in 2018 that she's a big meat eater and doesn't fill up on pasta or anything with added sugar, making her a good candidate for keto. Instead, she says she fills her plate with healthy fats, including avocado, coconut oil, and butter. (www.everydayhealth.com)

J-LO,51 years old launched this challenge on her Instagram account, she would spend ten days without ingesting sugars or carbohydrates and urged her followers to join the challenge to do it with her simultaneously. Its purpose has been none other than to get rid of junk food, eliminate sugar and reset your body by doing this 'detox cure'. (www.mujerhoy.com)

The secret of 50 years old Melissa McCarthy's transformative weight loss is a healthy diet, pure and simple. But not just any diet – it's a high-protein, low-carb diet, known as the Ketogenic Diet. (www.livin3.com)

Renee Zellweger, 51 years old actress. To lose the weight, Renee followed a high-protein low-carb diet and worked out for 2 hours each day. (www.hollandandbarrett.com)

Jennifer Aniston, 51 years old. The award-winning actress revealed that the 'Jennifer Aniston diet' consists six days a week she sticks to a gluten-free, low carb and high protein diet, then for one day of the week she eats whatever she wants! (www.womanmagazine.co.uk)

3. FAQ

What is the Keto Diet?

The Keto Diet is a nutritional strategy based on the reduction of carbohydrates, which forces the body to independently produce the glucose necessary for survival and to increase the energy consumption of the fats contained in the adipose tissue.

Why is it called Keto?

Ketogenic diet means "diet that produces ketone bodies" a metabolic residue of energy production. In the ketogenic diet the ketone bodies reach a level above the normal condition. The unwanted excess of ketone bodies, responsible for the tendency to lower blood pH, is called ketosis.

What to eat on the Keto Diet?

The most important aspect of achieving ketosis is to eat foods that do not contain carbohydrates, limit those that contain few and avoid foods that are rich in them.

Recommended foods are:

- *Meat, fish products and eggs*

- *Cheeses*

- *Fats and oils for seasoning*

- *Vegetables*

Not recommended foods are:

- *Cereals, potatoes and derivatives*

- *Legumes*

- *Fruits*

- *Sweet drinks, various sweets, beer, etc.*

Keto Diet & Menopause

During menopause, it can be more difficult for obese or overweight women to lose weight due to insulin resistance, for example. In this context, the application of a keto diet may therefore be useful in consideration of the increase in cardiovascular risks that characterize this phase of life.

Is Keto Diet Good For Women Over 50?

If you are a woman over 50, you may be more interested in losing weight than in your 30s. At this great age, many women experience a slow metabolism at a rate of about 50 calories a day.

Slowed metabolism coupled with less exercise, muscle degeneration, and the potential for increased cravings can make weight gain extremely difficult to control.

There are many diet options available to help you lose weight, but the keto diet has been one of the most popular lately.

Whether or not the Keto diet is right for you depends on a number of factors. Assuming you don't suffer from health problems, in general, a ketogenic diet can provide many benefits, especially for weight loss.

Recommendations

This book was written for recreational purposes only and the images of the recipes are for illustrative purposes only. It was not written by a doctor and is not a substitute for the advice of a nutritionist. Like any diet, ketogenic has positive and negative aspects. Starting a ketogenic diet requires constant supervision by your doctor.

4. KETO BREAKFAST RECIPES

1. Power Breakfast Omelete

Preparation Time: 5 minutes

Cooking Time: 5 minutes

Servings: 6

Nutrition: Carbs 2 grams, Protein 13 grams, Fats 29 grams, Calories 320

Ingredients:

- 1 cup Heavy cream
- 6 Eggs
- 5 Crispy slices of bacon
- 2 Chopped green onions
- 4 oz Cheddar cheese

Directions:

1. Warm the oven temperature to reach 350° F.
2. Whisk the eggs and seasonings.
3. Empty into the pie pan and top off with the remainder of the fixings.
4. Bake 30-35 minutes.
5. Wait for a few minutes before serving for the best results.

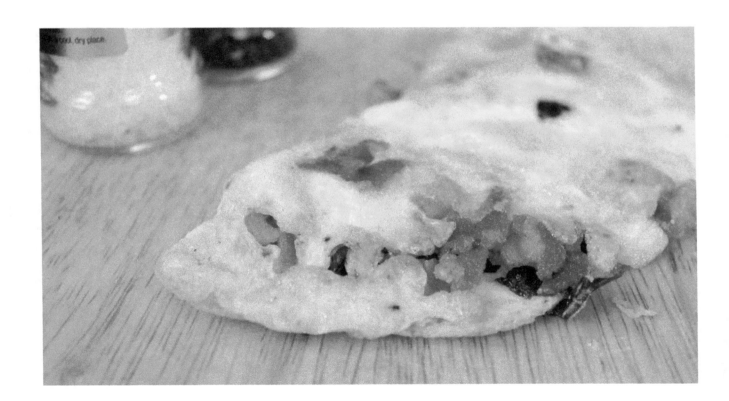

2. Fragola smoothie

Preparation Time: 5

Cooking Time: 15

Servings: 1

Nutrition: Carbs 5g, Protein 2g, Fats 16g, Calories 176

Ingredients:

- 5 medium strawberries, hulled
- 3 tablespoons heavy (whipping) cream
- 3 ice cubes
- Your favorite vanilla-flavored sweetener

Directions:

1. In a blender, combine all the ingredients and blend until smooth.
2. Enjoy right away!

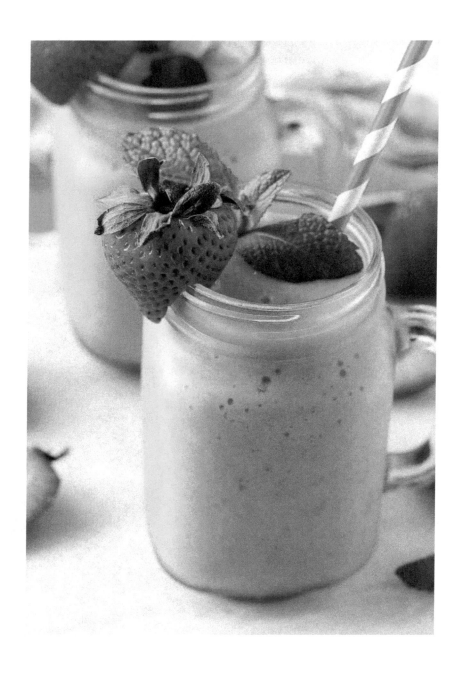

3. Women Power Bars

Preparation Time: 10 Minutes & Chill

Cooking Time: 20 minutes

Servings: 12

Nutrition: Carbs 4.5g, Protein 6.5g, Fats 22g, Fiber 2.5g, Calories 242

Ingredients:

- ½ cup pili nuts
- ½ cup whole hazelnuts
- ½ cup walnut halves
- ¼ cup hulled sunflower seeds
- ¼ cup unsweetened coconut flakes or chips
- ¼ cup hulled hemp seeds
- 2 tablespoons unsweetened cacao nibs
- 2 scoops collagen powder (I use 1 scoop Perfect Keto vanilla collagen and 1 scoop Perfect Keto unflavored collagen powder)
- ½ teaspoon ground cinnamon
- ½ teaspoon sea salt
- ¼ cup coconut oil, melted
- 1 teaspoon vanilla extract
- Stevia or monk fruit to sweeten (optional if you are using unflavored collagen powder)

Directions:

1. Line a 9-inch square baking pan with parchment paper.
2. In a food processor or blender, combine the pili nuts, hazelnuts, walnuts, sunflower seeds, coconut, hemp seeds, cacao nibs, collagen powder, cinnamon, and salt and pulse a few times.
3. Add the coconut oil, vanilla extract, and sweetener (if using).
4. Pulse again until the ingredients are combined. Do not over pulse or it will turn to mush. You want the nuts and seeds to still have some texture.
5. Pour the mixture into the prepared pan and press it into an even layer.
6. Cover with another piece of parchment (or fold over extra from the first piece) and place a heavy pan or dish on top to help press the bars together.
7. Refrigerate overnight and then cut into 12 bars.
8. Store the bars in individual storage bags in the refrigerator for a quick grab-and-go breakfast.

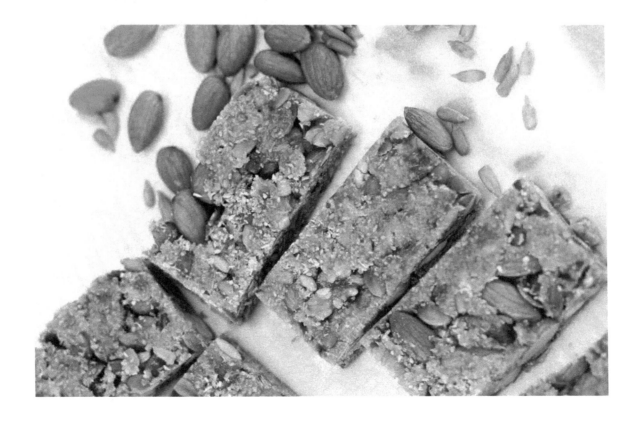

4. Wonder CheeseKeto

Preparation Time: 20 minutes

Cooking Time: 45 minutes

Servings: 24

Nutrition: Carbs 3g, Fats 12g, Protein 6g, Calories 152

Ingredients:

- Toppings
- 1/4 cup of mixed berries for each cheesecake, frozen and thawed
- Filling ingredients
- 1/2 teaspoon of vanilla extract
- 1/2 teaspoon of almond extract
- 3/4 cup of sweetener
- 6 eggs
- 8 ounces of cream cheese
- 16 ounces of cottage cheese
- Crust ingredients
- 4 tablespoons of salted butter
- 2 tablespoons of sweetener
- 2 cups of almonds, whole

Directions:

1. Preheat oven to around 350°F.
2. Pulse almonds in a food processor then add in butter and sweetener.
3. Pulse until all the ingredients mix well and a course dough forms.
4. Coat twelve silicone muffin pans using foil or paper liners.
5. Divide evenly the batter between the muffin pans then press into the bottom part until it forms a crust and bake for about 8 minutes.
6. In the meantime, mix in a food processor the cream cheese and cottage cheese then pulse until the mixture is smooth.
7. Put in the extracts and sweetener then combine until well mixed.
8. Add in eggs and pulse again until it becomes smooth; you might need to scrape down the mixture from the sides of the processor. Share equally the batter between the muffin pans, then bake for around 30-40 minutes until the middle is not wobbly when you shake lightly the muffin pan.
9. Put aside until cooled completely then put in the refrigerator for about 2 hours and then top with frozen and thawed berries.

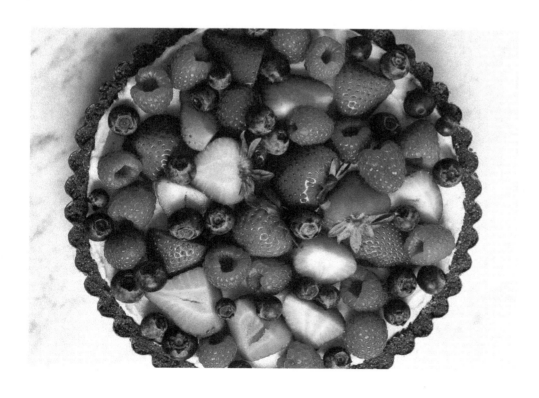

5. Roll Out the Bed

Preparation Time: 5 minutes

Cooking Time: 15 minutes

Servings: 5

Nutrition: 412.2 Calories 31.66 fats **2.26 carbs** 28.21 proteins

Ingredients:

- Non-stick cooking spray
- 5 patties of cooked breakfast sausage
- 5 slices of cooked bacon
- cups of cheddar cheese, shredded
- Pepper and salt
- 10 large eggs

Directions:

1. Preheat a skillet on medium to high heat then using a whisk, combine together two of the eggs in a mixing bowl.

2. After the pan has become hot, lower the heat to medium-low heat then put in the eggs. If you want to, you can utilize some cooking spray.

3. Season eggs with some pepper and salt.

4. Cover the eggs and leave them to cook for a couple of minutes or until the eggs are almost cooked.

5. Drizzle around 1/3 cup of cheese on top of the eggs then place a strip of bacon and divide the sausage into two and place on top.

6. Roll carefully the egg on top of the fillings. The roll up will almost look like a taquito. If you have a hard time folding over the egg, use a spatula to keep the egg intact until the egg have molded into a roll up.

7. Put aside the roll up then repeat the above steps until you have four more roll ups; you should have 5 roll ups in total.

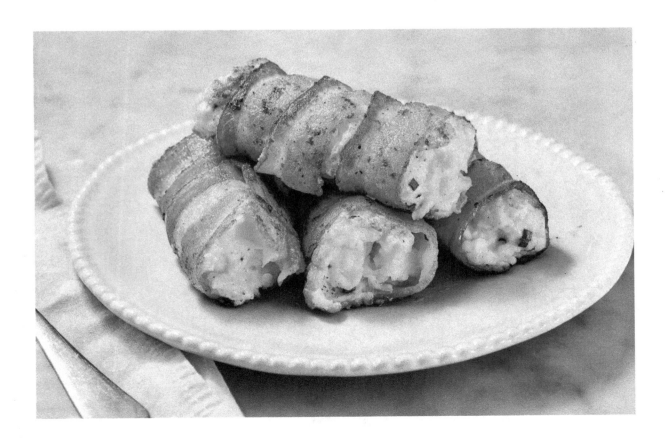

6. Green Way Smoothie

Preparation Time: 5 minutes

Cooking Time: -

Servings: 4

Nutrition: Calories 124, Fats 7.8g, **Carbs 2.9g**, Protein 3.2g

Ingredients:

- 6 kale leaves, chopped
- 3 stalks celery, chopped
- 1 ripe avocado, skinned and sliced
- 2 cups spinach, chopped
- 1 cucumber, peeled and chopped
- Chia seeds to garnish

Directions:

8. In a blender, add the kale, celery, avocado, and ice cubes, and blend for 45 seconds.
9. Add the spinach and cucumber, and process for another 45 seconds until smooth.
10. Pour the smoothie into glasses, garnish with chia seeds, and serve the drink immediately.

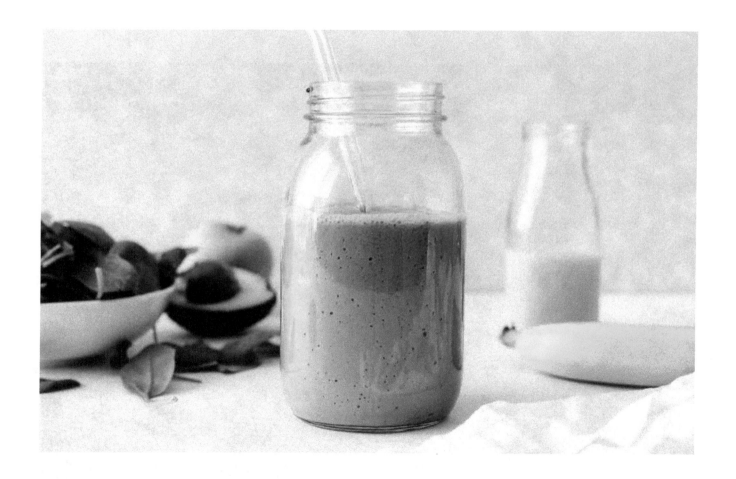

7. Spicy Muffin

Preparation Time: 10 minutes

Cooking Time: 20 minutes

Servings: 3

Nutrition: Calories 302, Fats 23.7g, **Carbs 3.2g**, Protein 20g

Ingredients:

- 2 heads broccoli, cut into small florets
- 2 red bell peppers, seeded and chopped
- ¼ cup chopped ham
- 2 teaspoon ghee
- 1 teaspoon dried oregano + extra to garnish
- Salt and black pepper to taste
- 8 fresh eggs

Directions:

1. Preheat oven to 425°F.
2. Melt the ghee in a frying pan over medium heat; brown the ham, stirring frequently, about 3 minutes.
3. Arrange the broccoli, bell peppers, and ham on a foil-lined baking sheet in a single layer, toss to combine; season with salt, oregano, and black pepper. Bake for 10 minutes until the vegetables have softened.
4. Remove, create eight indentations with a spoon, and crack an egg into each. Return to the oven and continue to bake for an additional 5 to 7 minutes until the egg whites are firm.
5. Season with salt, black pepper, and extra oregano, share the bake into four plates and serve with strawberry lemonade (optional).

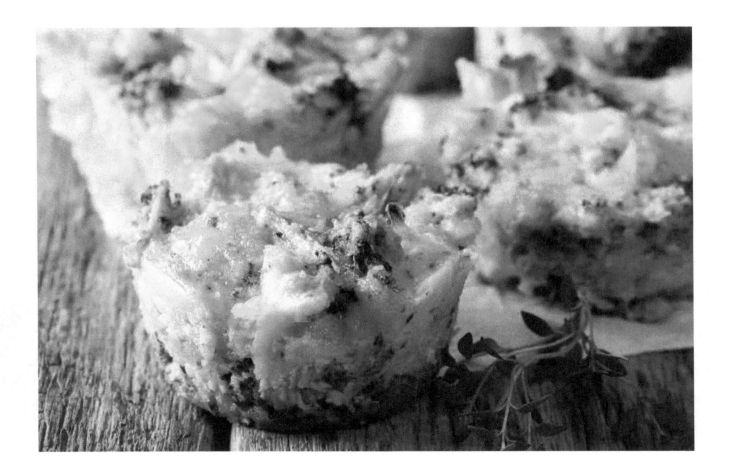

8. Keto DeliCookies

Preparation Time: 12 minutes

Cooking Time: 13 minutes

Servings: 8

Nutrition: 142 Calories, 13g Fats, **5g Carbs**, 3.5g Protein

Ingredients:

- 2 tablespoons coconut oil
- 1 tablespoon coconut milk
- 1 egg, whisked
- 1 cup coconut flour
- 1 cup almond flour
- 1 teaspoon baking powder
- 1/4 cup monk fruit powder
- 1 teaspoon pure anise extract
- 1/4 teaspoon ground cloves
- 1/2 teaspoon ground cinnamon
- A pinch of salt

Directions:

1. In a mixing bowl, beat the coconut oil, coconut milk, and egg. In a separate bowl, mix the flour, baking powder, monk fruit, anise extract, ground cloves, cinnamon, and salt.

2. Add the dry mixture to the wet mixture; mix to combine well. Shape the mixture into small balls and arrange them on a parchment-lined baking pan.

3. Bake at 360 degrees F for 13 minutes. Transfer to cooling racks for 10 minutes. Serve.

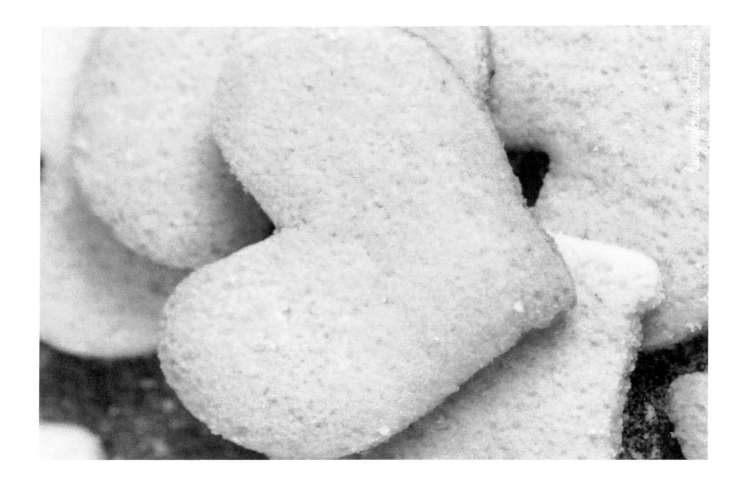

9. Sweet Bonjour Crepes

Preparation Time: 20 minutes

Coocking Time: 15 minutes

Servings: 4

Nutrition: Calories 330, Fats 21g, **Carbs 5g**, Protein 11g

Ingredients:

- 1 cup coconut flour
- 4 tbsp unsweetened cocoa powder
- 4 egg whites
- 1 cup + 4 tbsp flax milk
- 2 tbsp erythritol
- 2 tbsp olive oil

Caramel cream

- ½ cup salted butter
- 4 tbsp swerve brown sugar
- 1 tsp vanilla extract
- 1 cup heavy cream

Directions:

1. In a bowl, mix coconut flour and cocoa powder. In another bowl, whisk the egg whites, 1 cup flax milk, erythritol, and olive oil. Mix the wet ingredients with the dry ones until smooth.

2. Set a skillet over medium heat, grease with cooking spray, and pour in a ladleful of the batter. Swirl the pan quickly to spread the dough all around the skillet and cook the crepe for 2-3 minutes.

3. When it is firm enough to touch and cooked through, slide the crepe into a flat plate. Wipe the pan with a napkin and continue cooking until the remaining batter has finished. Put the butter and brown sugar in a pot and melt the butter over medium heat while stirring continually.

4. Keep cooking for 4 minutes after the butter has melted; be careful not to burn. Stir in the cream, reduce the heat to low, and let the sauce simmer for 10 minutes while stirring continually. Turn the heat off and stir in the vanilla extract. Once the crepes are ready, drizzle the caramel sauce over them, and serve.

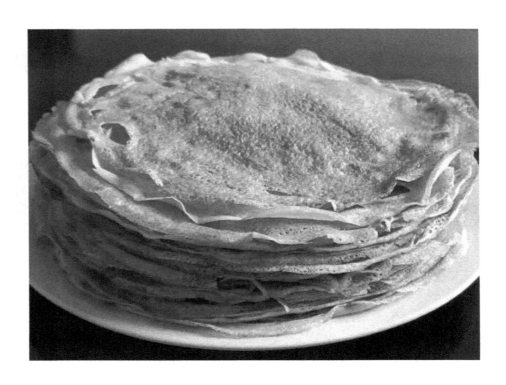

10. Greek Yogurt with Nut Granola

Preparation Time: 5 minutes

Cooking time: -

Servings: 4

Nutrition: Calories 361, Fats 31.2g, **Carbs 2g**, Protein 13g

Ingredients:
- 6 cups Greek yogurt
- 4 tbsp almond butter
- A handful toasted walnuts
- 3 tbsp unsweetened cocoa powder
- 4 tsp swerve brown sugar
- 2 cups nut granola for topping

Directions:
1. Combine the Greek yogurt, almond butter, walnuts, cocoa powder, and swerve brown sugar in a smoothie maker.
2. Puree at high speed until smooth and well mixed.
3. Share the smoothie into four breakfast bowls, top with a half cup of granola each one, and serve.

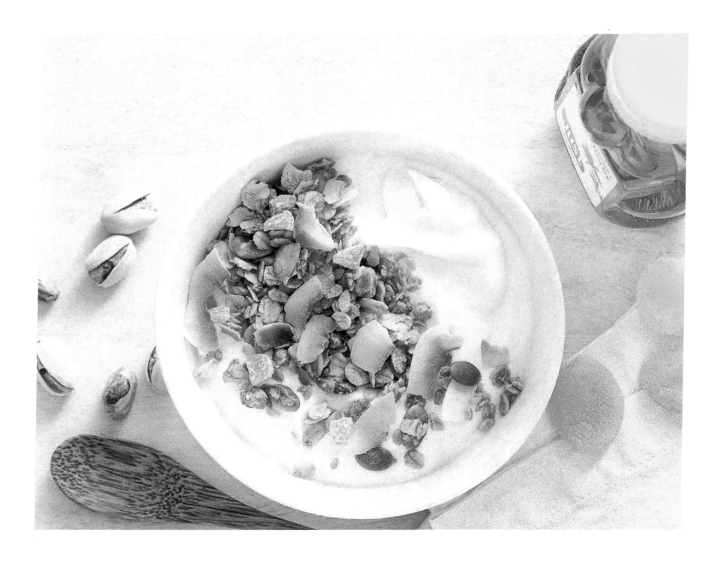

11. Protein Chocolate Shake

Preparation time: 5 minutes

Cooking time:-

Servings: 4

Nutrition: Calories 265, Fats 15.5g, Carbs 4g, Protein 12g

Ingredients:

- 3 cups flax milk, chilled
- 3 tsp unsweetened cocoa powder
- 1 medium avocado, peeled, sliced
- 1 cup coconut milk, chilled
- 3 mint leaves + extra to garnish
- 3 tbsp erythritol
- 1 tbsp low carb protein powder
- Whipping cream for topping

Directions:

1. Combine the flax milk, cocoa powder, avocado, coconut milk, 3 mint leaves, erythritol, and protein powder into the smoothie maker, and blend for 1 minute to smooth.

2. Pour the drink into serving glasses, lightly add some whipping cream on top, and garnish with 1 or 2 mint leaves.

3. Serve immediately

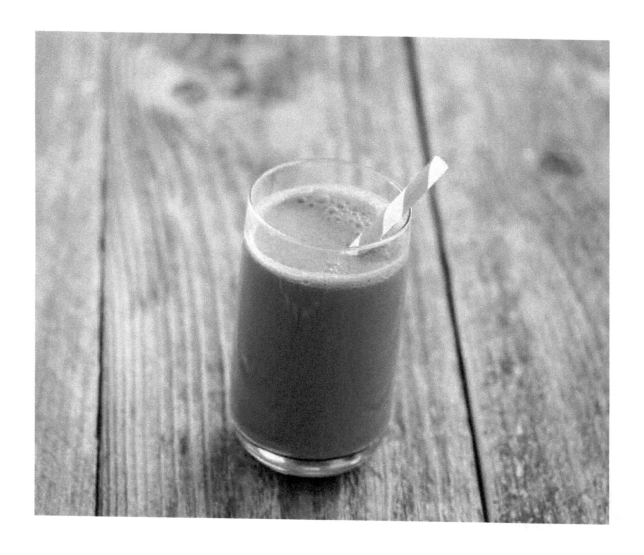

5. KETO LUNCH RECIPES

12. Spicy Chicken Wings

Preparation Time: 10 minutes

Cooking Time: 47 minutes

Servings: 3

Nutrition: Calories 391, **Carbs 1g,** Fats 33g, Protein: 31g

Ingredients:

- Hot sauce ¼ cup
- Coconut oil 4 tablespoons, plus more for rubbing on the wings
- Chicken wings 12 (fresh or frozen)
- Garlic 1 clove, minced
- Salt ¼ teaspoon
- Paprika ¼ teaspoon
- Cayenne pepper ¼ teaspoon
- Ground black pepper 1 dash

Directions:

1. Preheat your oven to 400 degrees F (200 degrees C).
2. Evenly spread chicken wings on a wire rack placed on a baking dish (it will save wings to become soggy on the bottom).
3. Rub each chicken wing with olive oil and season with salt and pepper, then bake for 45 minutes, or until crispy.
4. Meanwhile, in a saucepan combine coconut oil and garlic and cook over medium heat for 1 minute, or until fragrant.
5. Remove from heat and stir in hot sauce, salt, paprika, cayenne pepper and black pepper.
6. Remove wings from the oven and transfer to a large bowl.
7. Pour hot sauce mixture over wings and toss until each wing is coated with the sauce.
8. Serve immediately.

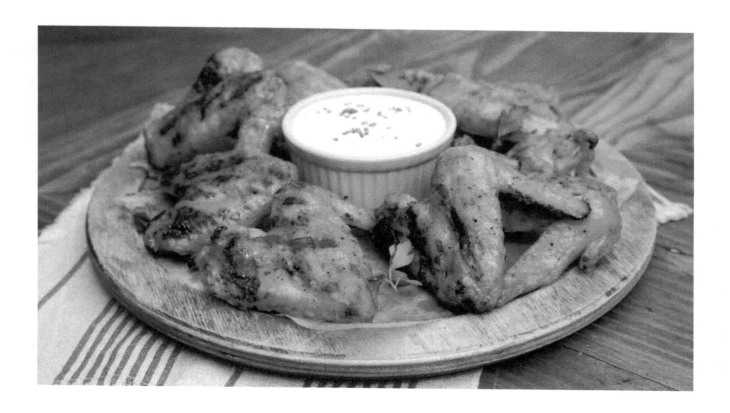

13. Caribbean Crispy Pork

Preparation Time: 15 minutes

Cooking Time: 4 minutes

Servings: 6

Nutrition: Calories 910.3, Protein 58.3g, **Carbs 5g**, Fats 69.6g

Ingredients:
- Five pounds pork shoulder
- Four tsp salt
- Two tsp. cumin
- One tsp. black pepper
- Two tbsps. oregano
- One red onion
- Four cloves garlic
- Orange juice
- Lemons juiced
- One-fourth cup of olive oil

Directions:
1. Rub the pork shoulder with salt in a bowl. Mix all the remaining items of the marinade in a blender.
2. Marinate the meat within eight hours. Cook within forty minutes. Warm-up your oven at 200 degrees. Roast the pork within thirty minutes.
3. Remove the meat juice. Simmer within twenty minutes. Shred the meat.
4. Pour the meat juice. Serve.

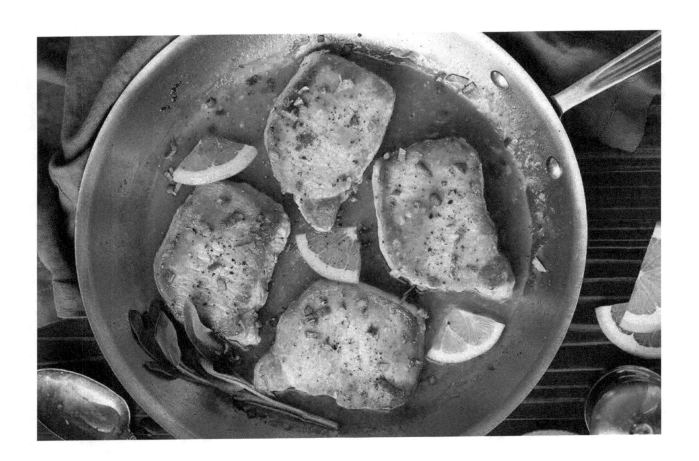

14. Frida Power Salad

Preparation Time: 7 minutes

Cooking Time: 10 minutes

Servings: 4

Nutrition: 220 Calories, **carbs: 2.8 g** fats 16.7 g, protein: 14.8 g.

Ingredients:

- 1 cup roasted chicken, shredded
- 1 bacon strip, cooked and chopped
- 1/2 medium avocado, chopped
- ¼ cup cheddar cheese, grated
- 1 hard-boiled egg, chopped
- 1 cup romaine lettuce, chopped
- 1 tablespoon. Olive oil
- 1 tablespoon. Apple cider vinegar
- Salt and pepper to taste

Directions:

1. Create the dressing by mixing apple cider vinegar, oil, salt and pepper.
2. Combine all the other Ingredients: in a mixing bowl.
3. Drizzle with the dressing and toss. Servings.
4. It can be refrigerated for up to 3 days.

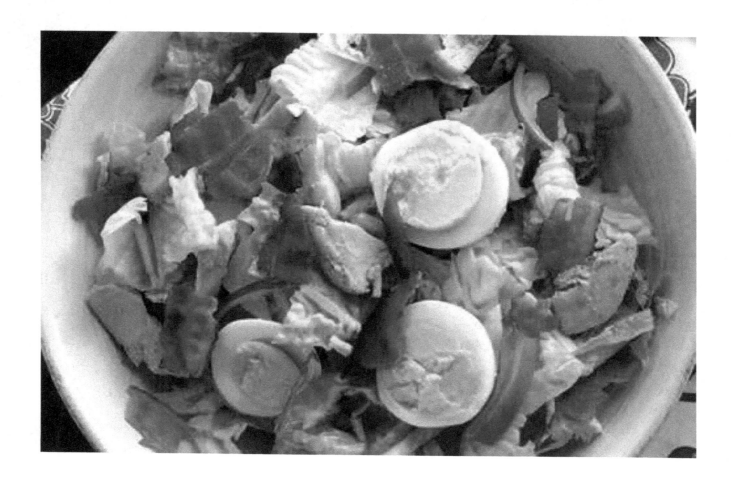

15. Incredible Fish and Ham Wrap

Preparation Time: 5 minutes

Cooking Time: 10 minutes

Servings: 3

Nutrition: 308 Calories, 19.9g Fats, **4.3g Carbs,** 27.8g Protein

Ingredients:

- 1/2 cup dry white wine
- 1/2 cup water
- 1/2 teaspoon mixed peppercorns
- 1/2 teaspoon dry mustard powder
- 1/2 pound ahi tuna steak
- 6 slices of ham
- 1/2 Hass avocado, peeled, pitted and sliced
- 1 tablespoon fresh lemon juice
- 6 lettuce leaves

Directions:

1. Add wine, water, peppercorns, and mustard powder to a skillet and bring to a boil. Add the tuna and simmer gently for 3 minutes to 5 minutes per side.
2. Discard the cooking liquid and slice tuna into bite-sized pieces. Divide the tuna pieces between slices of ham.
3. Add avocado and drizzle with fresh lemon. Roll the wraps up and place each wrap on a lettuce leaf. Serve well chilled.!

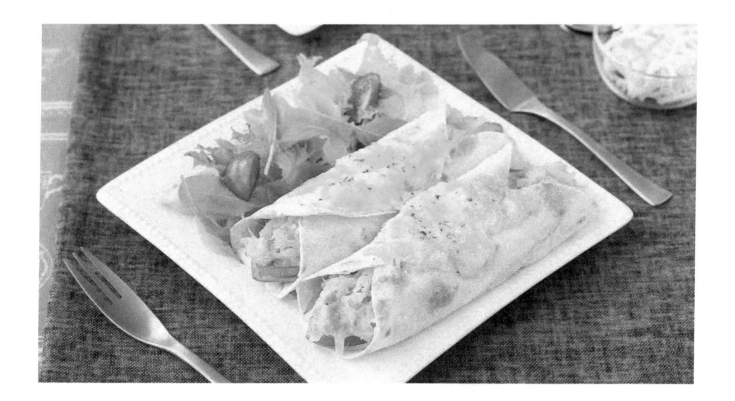

16. Marinated Glamour Salmon

Preparation Time: 40 minutes

Cooking Time: 10 minutes

Servings: 4

Nutrition: 331 Calories, 21.4g Fats, **2.2g Carbs**, 30.4g Protein

Ingredients:

- 4 (5-ounce) salmon steaks
- 2 cloves garlic, pressed
- 4 tablespoons olive oil
- 1 tablespoon Taco seasoning mix
- 2 tablespoons fresh lemon juice

Directions:

1. Place all of the above ingredients in a ceramic dish; cover and let it marinate for 40 minutes in your refrigerator.
2. Place the salmon steaks onto a lightly oiled grill pan; place under the grill for 6 minutes.
3. Turn them over and cook for a further 5 to 6 minutes, basting with the reserved marinade; remove from the grill.
4. Serve immediately and enjoy!

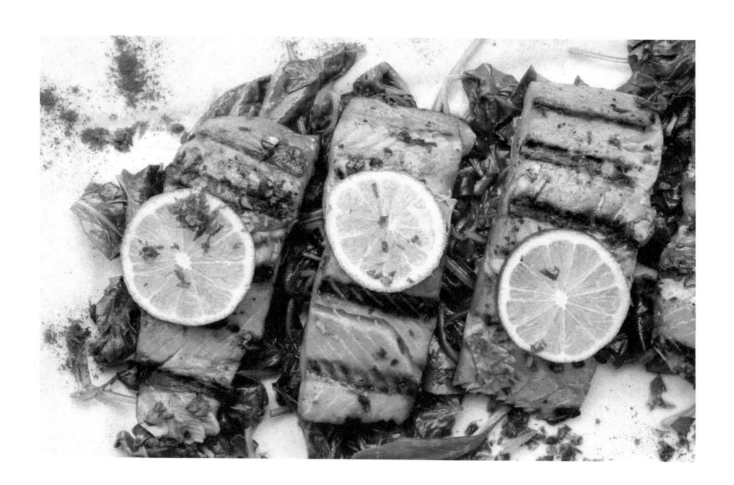

17. Grandma's meatballs

Preparation Time: 10 minutes

Cooking Time: 20 minutes

Servings: 4

Nutrition: Calories 454 **carbs: 5 g,** fat: 28.2 g, protein 43.2 g

Ingredients:

- 1 lb. Ground beef
- 1 egg, beaten
- Salt and pepper to taste
- 1 teaspoon garlic powder
- 1 teaspoon onion powder
- 2 tablespoons. Butter
- ¼ cup mayonnaise
- ¼ cup pickled jalapeños
- 1 cup cheddar cheese, grated

Directions:

1. Combine the cheese, mayonnaise, pickled jalapenos, salt, pepper, garlic powder and onion powder in a large mixing bowl.
2. Add the beef and egg and combine using clean hands.
3. Form large meatballs makes about 12.
4. Fry the meatballs in the butter over medium heat for about 4 minutes on each side or until golden brown.
5. Servings warm with a keto-friendly side.
6. The meatball mixture can also be used to make a meatloaf. Just preheat your oven to 400 degrees f, press the mixture into a loaf pan and bake for about 30 minutes or until the top is golden brown.
7. It can be refrigerated for up to 5 days or frozen for up to 3 months.

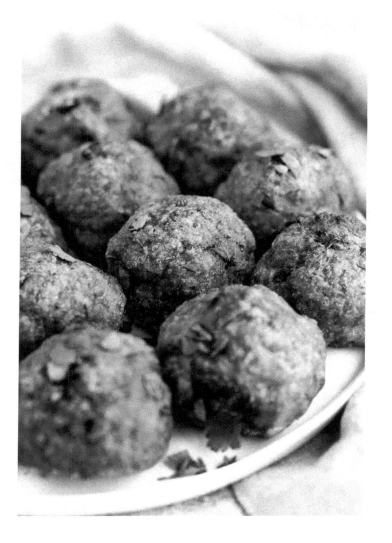

18. Very Simple Keto Chicken

Preparation Time: 15 minutes

Cooking Time: 1 hour & 30 minutes

Servings: 2

Nutrition: calories 980.3, protein: 57.2g, **carbs: 0.4g**, fats 81.3g

Ingredients:

- Three pounds whole chicken
- Pepper and salt
- Two tsp. Barbecue seasoning
- Five ounces butter
- One lemon
- Two onions
- One-fourth cup water
- One tsp. Butter

Directions:

1. Warm-up oven at 170 degrees. Grease the baking dish.
2. Rub the chicken with pepper, salt, and barbecue seasoning. Put in the baking dish.
3. Arrange lemon wedges and onions surrounding the chicken put slices of butter.
4. Bake within 1 hour and 30 minutes. Slice and serve.

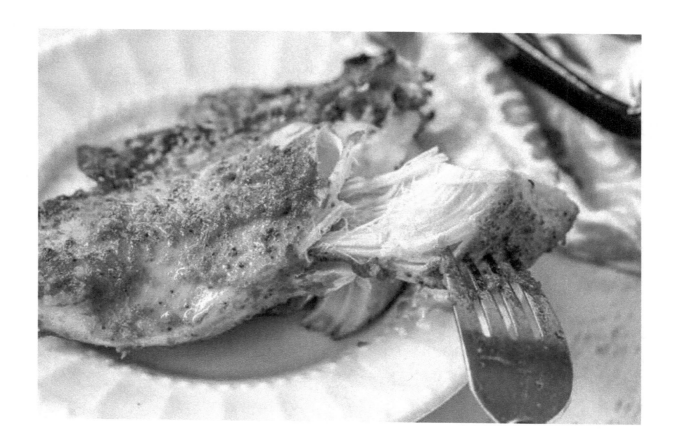

19. Popeye Spinach Chicken

Preparation Time: 10 minutes

Cooking Time: 35 minutes

Servings: 4

Nutrition: Calories 340, Fats 30.2g, **Carbs 3.1g**, Protein 15g

Ingredients:

- 1 lb chicken breasts
- 1 tsp mixed spice seasoning
- Pink salt and black pepper to taste
- 2 loose cups baby spinach
- 3 tsp olive oil
- 4 oz cream cheese
- 1 ¼ cups mozzarella cheese, grated
- 4 tbsp water

Directions:

1. Preheat oven to 370°F. Season chicken with spice mix, salt, and black pepper.
2. Pat with your hands to have the seasoning stick on the chicken.
3. Put in the casserole dish and layer spinach over the chicken.
4. Mix the oil with cream cheese, mozzarella, salt, and pepper and stir in water a tablespoon at a time.
5. Pour the mixture over the chicken and cover the casserole dish with aluminium foil. Bake for 20 minutes.
6. Remove the foil and continue cooking for 15 minutes until a nice golden brown color is formed on top.
7. Take out and allow sitting for 5 minutes. Serve warm with braised asparagus.

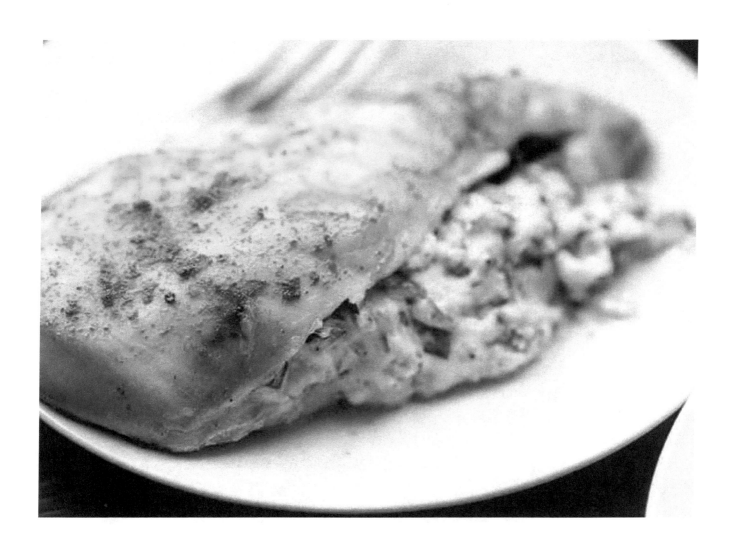

20. Tuna Thai

Preparation Time: 5 minutes

Cooking Time: 20 minutes

Servings: 4

Nutrition: 389 Calories, 17.9g Fats, **3.5g Carbs,** 50.3g Protein

Ingredients:

- 1 tablespoon peanut oil
- 4 tuna fillets
- 1 teaspoon freshly grated ginger
- Kosher salt and freshly ground black pepper, to taste
- 1 teaspoon cayenne pepper
- 1/2 teaspoon cumin seeds
- 1/4 teaspoon ground cinnamon

Sauce:

- 2 scallions, chopped
- 2 garlic cloves, minced
- 1 tablespoon fresh cilantro, chopped
- 1 teaspoon Sriracha sauce
- 4 tablespoons mayonnaise
- 1/2 cup sour cream
- 1 teaspoon stone-ground mustard

Directions:

1. Preheat your oven to 375 degrees F. Line a baking sheet with foil.

2. Place the tuna fillets onto the prepared baking sheet; now, fold up all 4 sides of the foil. Add peanut oil, grated ginger, salt, black pepper, cayenne pepper, cumin, and cinnamon.

3. Fold the sides of the foil over the fish fillets, sealing the packet. Bake until cooked through, approximately 20 minutes.

4. To make the sauce, whisk together all of the sauce ingredients. Serve immediately and enjoy!

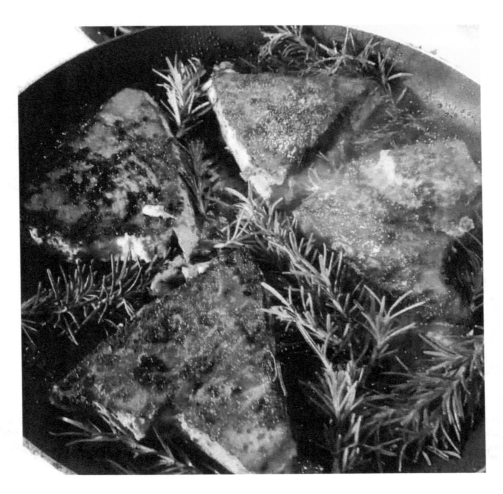

21. Italian Parmesano & Yogurt Wings

Preparation Time: 5 minutes

Cooking Time: 20 minutes

Servings: 6

Nutrition: Calories 452, Fats 36.4g, **Carbs 4g**, Protein 24g

Ingredients:
- 1 cup Greek-style yogurt
- 2 tbsp extra-virgin olive oil
- 1 tbsp fresh dill, chopped
- 2 lb chicken wings
- Salt and black pepper to taste
- ½ cup butter, melted
- ½ cup hot sauce
- ¼ cup Parmesan cheese, grated

Directions:
1. Preheat oven to 400°F.
2. Mix yogurt, olive oil, dill, salt, and black pepper in a bowl.
3. Chill while making the chicken.
4. Season wings with salt and pepper.
5. Line them on a baking sheet and grease with cooking spray.
6. Bake for 20 minutes until golden brown.
7. Mix butter, hot sauce, and Parmesan cheese in a bowl.
8. Toss chicken in the sauce to evenly coat and plate.
9. Serve with yogurt dipping sauce.

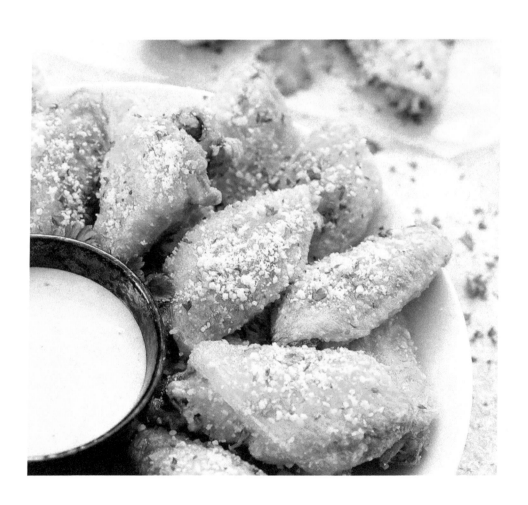

22. Bass & Pepper

Preparation Time: 5 minutes

Cooking Time: 15 minutes

Servings: 6

Nutrition: 227 Calories, 8.3g Fats, **4.8g Carbs**, 32.3g Protein

Ingredients:

- 2 tablespoons butter, at room temperature
- 1 leek, chopped
- 1 bell pepper, chopped
- 1 serrano pepper, chopped
- 2 garlic cloves, minced
- 2 tablespoons fresh coriander, chopped
- 2 vine-ripe tomatoes, pureed
- 4 cups fish stock
- 2 pounds sea bass fillets, chopped into small chunks
- 1 tablespoon Old Bay seasoning
- 1/2 teaspoon sea salt, to taste
- 2 bay laurels

Directions:

1. Melt the butter in a heavy-bottomed pot over moderate heat. Stir in the leek and peppers and sauté them for about 5 minutes or until tender.
2. Stir in the garlic and continue to sauté for 30 to 40 seconds more.
3. Add in the remaining ingredients; gently stir to combine. Turn the heat to medium-low and partially cover the pot.
4. Now, let it cook until thoroughly heated, approximately 10 minutes longer. Lastly, discard the bay laurels and serve warm. Enjoy!

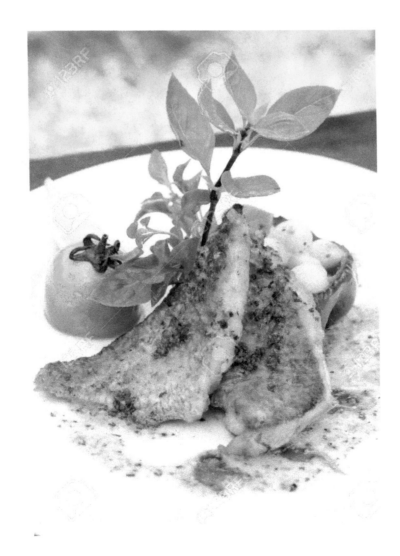

23. Burger in Italy

Preparation Time: 10 minutes

Cooking Time: 12 minutes

Servings: 4

Nutrition: calories 441, fats 37g, protein 22g, **carbs 4g**

Ingredients:

- 1 pound 75% lean ground beef
- 1/4 cup ground almonds
- 2 tbsp. Chopped fresh basil
- 1 tsp. Minced garlic
- 1/4 tsp. Sea salt
- 1 tbsp. Olive oil
- 1 tomato cut into 4 thick slices
- 1/4 sweet onion, sliced thinly

Directions:

1. 1. In a medium bowl, mix together the ground beef, ground almonds, basil, garlic, and salt until well mixed.
2. 2.Form the beef mixture into four equal patties and flatten them to about 1/2 inch thick.
3. 3.Place a large skillet on medium-high heat and add the olive oil.
4. 4.Panfry the burgers until cooked through, flipping them once, about 12 minutes in total.
5. 5.Pat away excess grease with a paper towel and serve the burgers with a slice of tomato and onion.

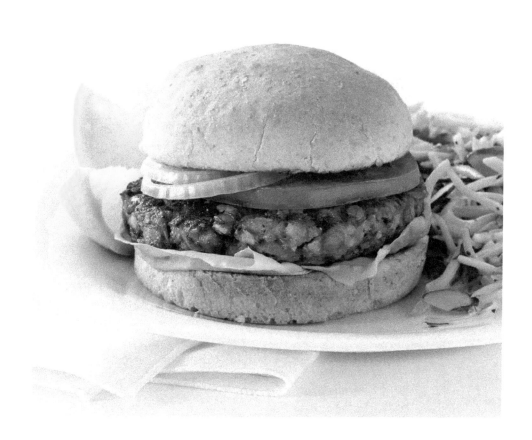

24. Blue Bacon Eggs

Preparation Time: 10 minutes

Cooking Time: 90-120 minutes

Servings: 3

Nutrition: Calories 217, Fats 16 g, **Carbs 1 g**, Protein 6 g

Ingredients:

- 8 eggs
- ¼ cup crumbled bleu cheese
- 3 slices of cooked bacon
- ¼ cup sour cream
- 1/3 cup mayo
- ¼ tsp. pepper and dill
- ½ tsp. salt
- 1 tbsp. mustard
- parsley

Directions:

1. Hard boil your eggs and then cut them half. Place the yolks in a bowl.
2. With a fork, mash the yolks, add the sour cream, mayo, bleu cheese, mustard, and the seasoning and mix until creamy enough for your taste.
3. Slice up the bacon to small pieces.
4. Stir in the rest of the ingredients and fill up the eggs.
5. Serve and enjoy!

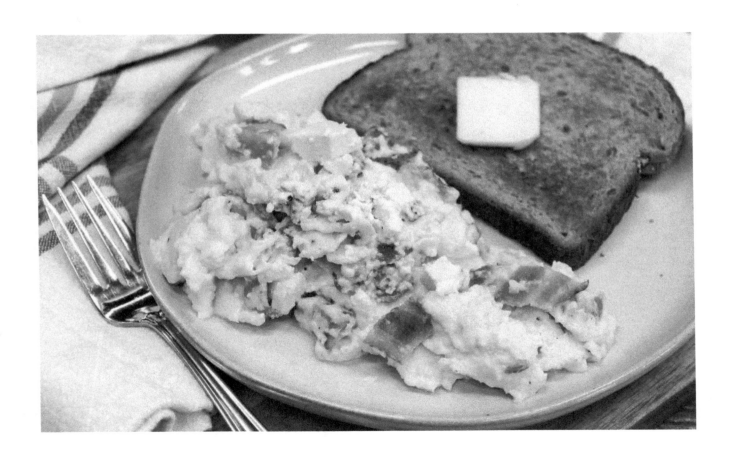

25. Mediterranean Lamb Chops

Preparation Time: 10 minutes

Cooking Time: 6 minutes

Servings: 4

Nutrition: calories 457, protein 63g, fats 9g, **carbs 4g**

Ingredients:
- 1 tbsp. Black pepper
- 1 tbsp. Dried oregano
- 1 tbsp. Minced garlic
- 2 tbsp. Lemon juice
- 2 tsp. Olive oil
- 2 tsp. Seal salt
- 8 pieces of lamb loin chops, around 4 ounces

Directions:
1. 1.In a big bowl or dish, combine the black pepper, salt, minced garlic, lemon juice and oregano.
2. Then rub it equally on all sides of the lamb chops.
3. 2.Then place a skillet on high heat. After a minute, coat skillet with the cooking spray and place the lamb chops in the skillet. Sear chops for a minute on each side.
4. 3.Lower heat to medium; continue cooking chops for 2 -3 minutes per side until desired doneness is reached
5. 4.Let the chops rest for five minutes before serving.

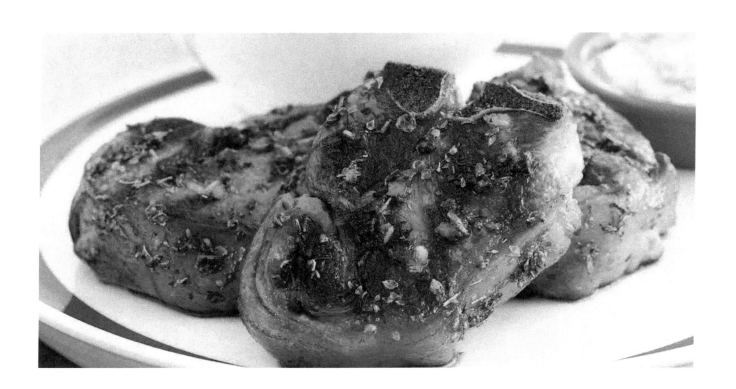

6. KETO DINNER RECIPES

26. LowCarb Chicken Peanut

Preparation Time: 1 hour

Cooking Time: 15 minutes

Servings: 6

Nutrition: Calories 492, Fats 36g, **Carbs 3g**, Protein 35g

Ingredients:

Chicken ingredients
- 1 tbsp wheat-free soy sauce
- 1 tbsp sugar-free fish sauce
- 1 tbsp lime juice
- 1 tsp cilantro, chopped
- 1 minced garlic
- 1 tsp minced ginger
- 1 tbsp olive oil
- 1 tbsp rice wine vinegar
- 1 tsp cayenne pepper
- 1 tbsp erythritol
- 6 chicken thighs

Peanut sauce
- ½ cup peanut butter
- 1 tsp minced garlic
- 1 tbsp lime juice
- 2 tbsp water
- 1 tsp minced ginger
- 1 tbsp jalapeño pepper, chopped
- 2 tbsp rice wine vinegar
- 2 tbsp erythritol
- 1 tbsp fish sauce

Directions:

1. Combine all chicken ingredients in a large Ziploc bag.
2. Seal the bag and shake to combine. Refrigerate for 1 hour.
3. Remove from the fridge about 15 minutes before cooking. Preheat the grill to medium heat.
4. Cook the chicken for 7 minutes per side until golden brown.
5. Remove to a serving plate. Whisk together all the sauce ingredients in a mixing bowl.
6. Serve the chicken drizzled with peanut sauce.

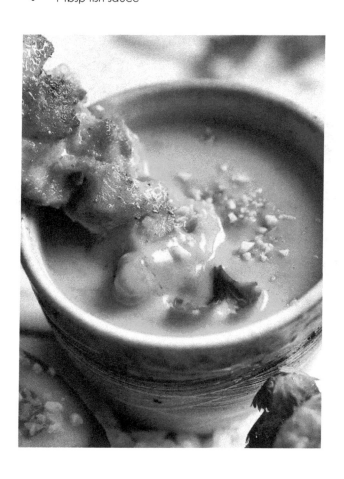

27. Salmon Fillets with Marsala Wine

Preparation Time: 5 minutes

Cooking Time: 15 minutes

Servings: 6

Nutrition: Calories 18.5g, Fats, **4g Carbs**, 39.9g Protein

Ingredients:

- 2 tablespoons peanut oil
- 2 bell peppers, deseeded and sliced
- 1/2 cup scallions, chopped
- 2 cloves garlic, minced
- 4 tablespoons Marsala wine
- 2 ripe tomatoes, pureed
- 2 ½ pounds salmon fillets
- Sea salt and ground black pepper, to taste
- 1/4 teaspoon ground bay leaf
- 1 teaspoon paprika

Directions:

1. Heat the peanut oil in a large frying pan over a moderate flame. Now, sauté the bell peppers and scallions for 3 minutes.

2. Add in the garlic and continue to sauté for 30 seconds more or until aromatic but not until it's browned.

3. Add a splash of wine to deglaze the pan. Stir in the remaining ingredients and turn the heat to simmer.

4. Let it cook, partially covered, for 15 minutes or until the salmon is cooked through.

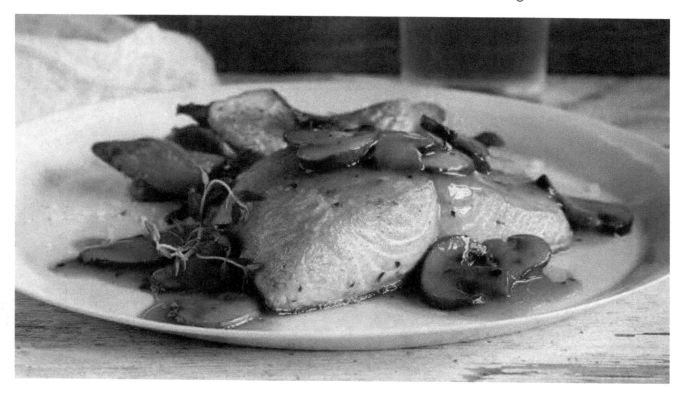

28. Delicious Stuffed Chicken

Preparation Time: 20 minutes

Cooking Time: 30 minutes

Servings: 4

Nutrition: Calories 491, Fats 36g, **Carbs 3.5g**, Protein 38g

Ingredients:

- 4 chicken breasts
- ½ cup mozzarella cheese, grated
- ⅓ cup Parmesan cheese
- 6 oz cream cheese, softened
- 2 cups spinach, chopped
- ½ tsp ground nutmeg

Breading

- 2 eggs
- ⅓ cup almond flour
- 2 tbsp olive oil
- ½ tsp parsley
- ⅓ cup Parmesan cheese
- 1 tsp onion powder

Directions:

1. Pound the chicken until it doubles in size.
2. Mix the cream cheese, spinach, mozzarella cheese, nutmeg, salt, black pepper, and Parmesan cheese in a bowl.
3. Divide the mixture between the chicken breasts.
4. Close the chicken around the filling. Wrap the breasts with cling film.
5. Refrigerate for 15 minutes.
6.
7. Preheat oven to 370°F. Beat the eggs in a shallow dish.
8. Combine all other breading ingredients in a bowl.
9. Dip the chicken in egg first, then in the breading mixture.
10. Heat the olive oil in a pan over medium heat. Cook chicken for 3-5 minutes on all sides. Transfer to a baking sheet.
11. Bake for 20 minutes. Serve.

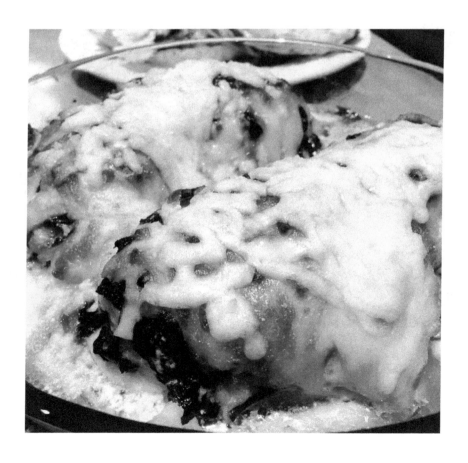

29. Green Noodles & Feta

Preparation Time: 15 minutes

Cooking Time: 15 minutes

Servings: 1

Nutrition: Carbs 5 grams, Protein 4 grams, Fats 8 grams, Calories 105

Ingredients:

- Quartered plum tomato 1
- Spiralized zucchini 2
- Feta cheese 8 cubes
- Pepper 1 tsp.
- Olive oil 1 tbsp.

Directions:

1. Set the oven temperature to reach 375° Fahrenheit.
2. Slice the noodles with a spiralizer and put the olive oil, tomatoes, pepper, and salt.
3. Bake within 10 to 15 minutes. Transfer then put cheese cubes, toss. Serve.

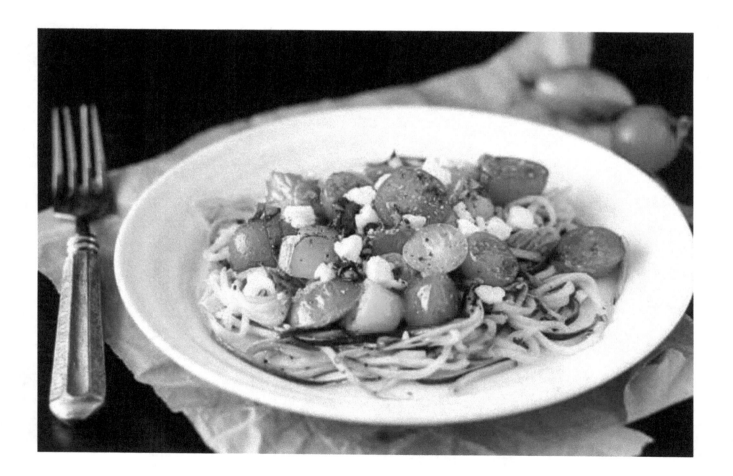

30. Chicken with Fashion Sauce

Preparation Time: 10 minutes

Cooking Time: 30 minutes

Servings: 4

Nutrition: Calories 345, Fats 12g, **Carbs 4g**, Protein 24g

Ingredients:

- 1 ½ chicken thighs
- Salt and black pepper to taste
- 2 shallots, chopped
- 2 tbsp canola oil
- 4 pancetta strips, chopped
- 2 garlic cloves, minced
- 10 oz white mushrooms, halved
- 1 cup white wine
- 1 cup whipping cream

Directions:

1. Warm the canola oil a pan over medium heat.
2. Cook the pancetta for 3 minutes.
3. Add in the chicken, sprinkle with pepper and salt, and cook until brown, about 5 minutes.
4. Remove to a plate. In the same pan, sauté shallots, mushrooms, and garlic for 6 minutes.
5. Return the pancetta and chicken to the pan.
6. Stir in the white wine and 1 cup of water and bring to a boil.
7. Reduce the heat and simmer for 20 minutes.
8. Pour in the whipping cream and warm without boiling.
9. Serve with steamed asparagus.

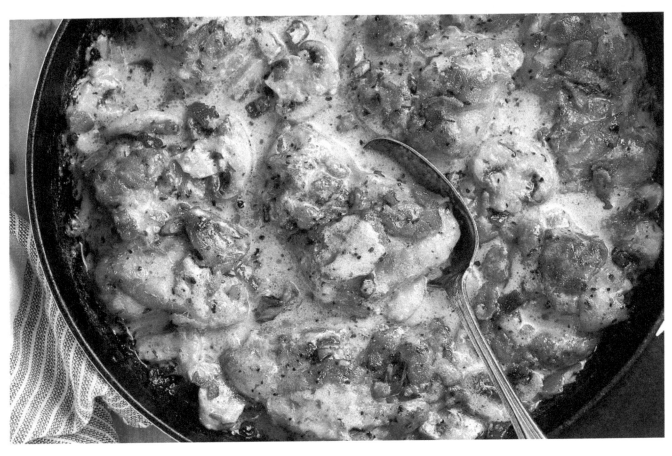

31. Keto Sprouts

Preparation Time: 15 minutes

Cooking Time: 40 minutes

Servings: 6

Nutrition: Carbs 3.9 g, Protein 7.9 g, Fats 6.9 g, Calories 113

Ingredients:
- Bacon (16 oz.)
- Brussels sprouts (16 oz.)
- Black pepper

Directions:
1. Warm the oven to reach 400° Fahrenheit.
2. Slice the bacon into small lengthwise pieces. Put the sprouts and bacon with pepper.
3. Bake within 35 to 40 minutes.
4. Serve.

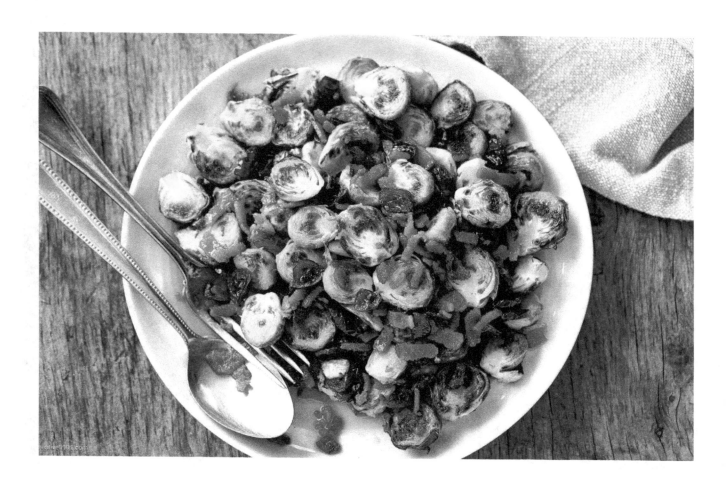

32. Carp Fillet with Coconut Milk

Preparation Time: 10 minutes

Cooking Time: 5 minutes

Servings: 3

Nutrition: 443 Calories, 28.3g Fats, **2.6g Carbs**, 42.5g Protein

Ingredients:

- 3 carp fillets
- 1 teaspoon chili powder
- 1 teaspoon cumin powder
- 1 teaspoon turmeric powder
- 1 coriander powder
- 1/2 teaspoon garam masala
- 1/2 teaspoon flaky salt
- 1/4 teaspoon cayenne pepper
- 3 tablespoons full-fat coconut milk
- 1 egg
- 2 tablespoons olive oil
- 6 curry leaves, for garnish

Directions:

1. Pat the fish fillets with kitchen towels and add to a large resealable bag.
2. Add the spices to the bag and shake to coat on all sides.
3. In a shallow dish, whisk the coconut milk and egg until frothy and well combined.
4. Dip the fillets into the egg mixture.
5. Then, heat the oil in a large frying pan.
6. Fry the fish fillets on both sides until they are cooked through and the coating becomes crispy.
7. Serve with curry leaves and enjoy!

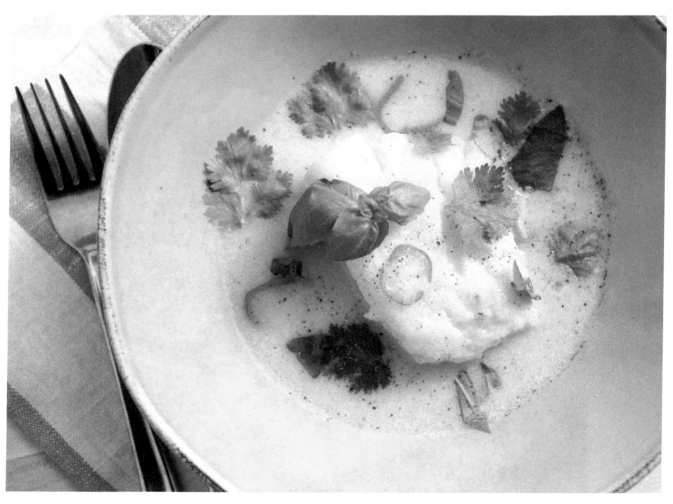

33. Espresso Pork BBQ

Preparation Time: 15 minutes

Cooking Time: 60 minutes

Servings: 4

Nutrition: Carbs 2.6 g, Protein 24 g, Fats 68 g, Calories 644

Ingredients:
- Beef stock 1.5 cups
- Pork belly 2 lb.
- Olive oil 4 tbsp)
- Low-carb barbecue dry rub
- Instant Espresso Powder 2 tbsp.

Directions:
1. Set the oven at 350° Fahrenheit.
2. Heat-up the beef stock in a small saucepan.
3. Mix in the dry barbecue rub and espresso powder.
4. Put the pork belly, skin side up in a shallow dish and drizzle half of the oil over the top.
5. Put the hot stock around the pork belly. Bake within 45 minutes.
6. Sear each slice within three minutes per side. Serve.

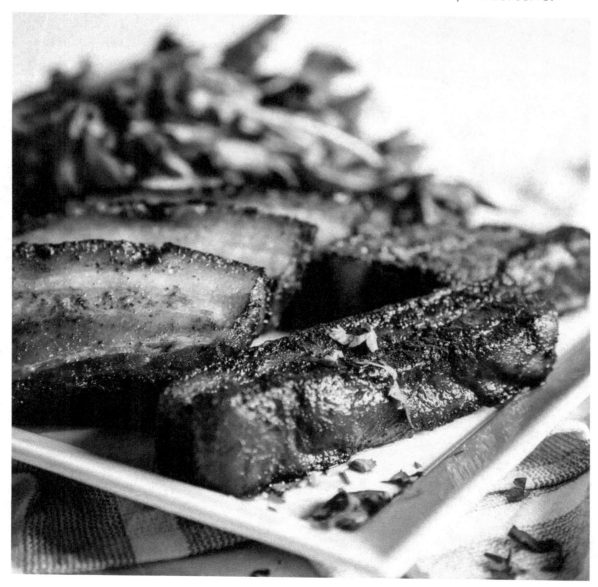

34. Keto Kebab

Preparation Time: 1 hour

Cooking Time: 5 minutes

Servings: 6

Nutrition: Calories 198, Fats, 13.5g, **Carbs 3.1g**, Protein 17.5g

Ingredients:

- 2 lb chicken breasts, cubed
- 3 tbsp sesame oil
- 1 cup red bell peppers, chopped
- 2 tbsp five-spice powder
- 2 tbsp granulated sweetener
- 1 tbsp fish sauce

Directions:

1. Combine the sesame oil, fish sauce, five-spice powder, and granulated sweetener in a bowl and mix well.
2. Add in the chicken and toss to coat.
3. Let marinate for 1 hour in the fridge.
4. Preheat the grill. Thread the chicken and bell peppers onto skewers.
5. Grill for 3 minutes per side.
6. Serve warm with steamed broccoli.

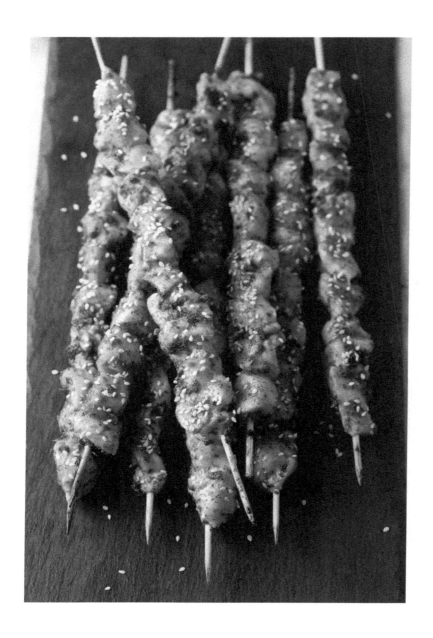

35. Hungarian Halászlé

Preparation Time: 10 minutes

Cooking Time: 10 minutes

Servings: 2

Nutrition: 252 Calories, 12.6g Fats, **5g Carbs**, 28.2g Protein

Ingredients:

- 1 tablespoon canola oil
- 2 bell peppers, chopped
- 1 Hungarian wax pepper, chopped
- 1 garlic clove, minced
- 1 red onion, chopped
- 1/2 pound tilapia, cut into bite-sized pieces
- 1 ½ cups fish broth
- 2 vine-ripe tomatoes, pureed
- 1 teaspoon sweet paprika
- 1/2 teaspoon mixed peppercorns, crushed
- 1 bay laurel
- 1/2 teaspoon sumac
- 1/2 teaspoon dried thyme
- 1/4 teaspoon dried rosemary
- Kosher salt, to season
- 1/2 teaspoon garlic, minced
- 2 tablespoons sour cream

Directions:

1. Heat the canola oil in a Dutch oven over medium-high heat. Now, sauté the peppers, garlic, and onion until tender and aromatic.

2. Now, stir in the tilapia, broth, tomatoes, and spices. Reduce the heat to medium-low. Let it simmer, covered, for 9 to 13 minutes.

3.

4. Meanwhile, mix 1/2 teaspoon of minced garlic with the sour cream. Serve with the warm paprikash and enjoy!

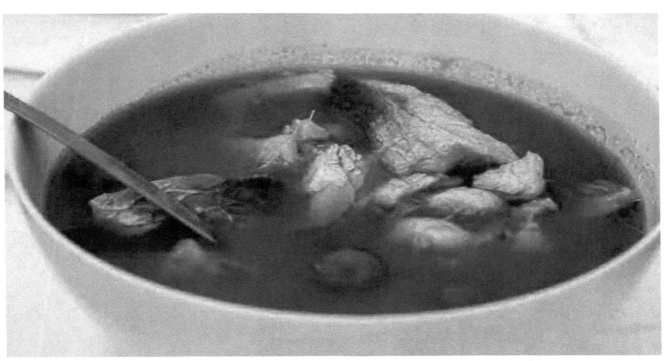

7. KETO SNACK RECIPES

36. Yellow Caribbean Waffles

Preparation Time: 30 minutes

Cooking Time: 30 minutes

Servings: 4

Nutrition: Carbs 4g, Fats 13g, Protein 5g, Calories 155

Ingredients:

- 4 eggs
- 1 ripe banana
- ¾ cup coconut milk
- ¾ cup almond flour
- 1 pinch of salt
- 1 tbsp. of ground psyllium husk powder
- 1/2 tsp. vanilla extract
- 1 tsp. baking powder
- 1 tsp. of ground cinnamon
- Butter or coconut oil for frying

Directions:

1. Mash the banana thoroughly until you get a mashed potato consistency.
2. Add all the other Ingredients in and whisk thoroughly to evenly distribute the dry and wet Ingredients. You should be able to get a pancake-like consistency
3. Fry the waffles in a pan or use a waffle maker.
4. You can serve it with hazelnut spread and fresh berries. Enjoy!

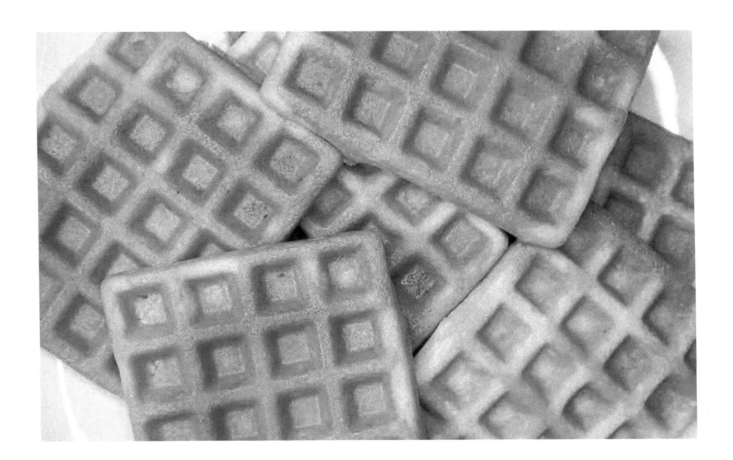

37. High Protein Granola

Preparation Time: 30 minutes

Cooking Time: 40 minutes

Servings: 12

Nutrition: Carbs 4,7g, Fats 23g, Protein 6g, Calories 247

Ingredients:

- 1 cup shredded coconut or almond flour
- 1 1/2 cups almonds
- 1 1/2 cups pecans
- 1/3 cup swerve sweetener
- 1/3 cup vanilla whey protein powder
- 1/3 cup peanut butter
- 1/4 cup sunflower seeds
- 1/4 cup butter
- 1/4 cup water

Directions:

1. Preheat the oven to 300 degrees Fahrenheit and prepare a baking sheet with parchment paper
2. Place the almonds and pecans in a food processor. Put them all in a large bowl and add the sunflower seeds, shredded coconut, vanilla, sweetener, and protein powder.
3. Melt the peanut butter and butter together in the microwave.
4. Mix the melted butter in the nut mixture and stir it thoroughly until the nuts are well-distributed.
5. Put in the water to create a lumpy mixture.
6. Scoop out small amounts of the mixture and place it on the baking sheet.
7. Bake for 30 minutes. Enjoy!

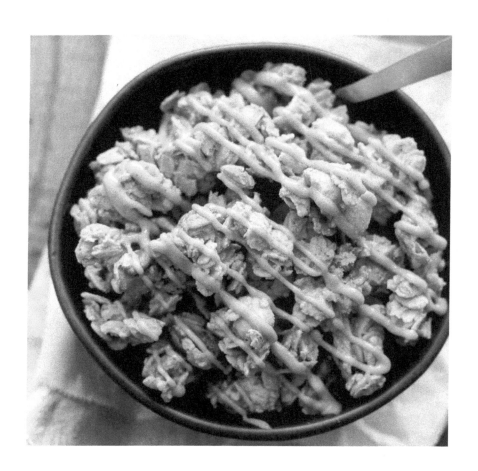

38. Keto Nachos

Preparation Time: 30 minutes

Cooking Time: 20 minutes

Servings: 2

Nutrition: 280 calories, 21.8 fats, 18.6g protein, **2.44g carbs**

Ingredients:

- 1/2 cup shredded Swiss cheese
- 1/2 cup shredded cheddar cheese
- 1/8 cup cooked bacon pieces

Directions:

1. Preheat the oven to 300 degrees Fahrenheit and prepare the baking sheet by lining it with parchment paper.
2. Start by spreading the Swiss cheese on the parchment. Sprinkle it with bacon and then top it off again with the cheese.
3. Bake until the cheese has melted. This should take around 10 minutes or less.
4. Allow the cheese to cool before cutting them into triangle strips.
5. Grab another baking sheet and place the triangle cheese strips on top. Broil them for 2 to 3 minutes so they'll get chunky.

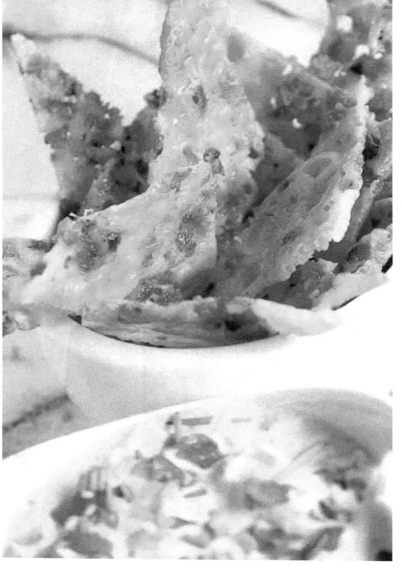

39. Keto Fried Beans

Preparation Time: 10 minutes

Cooking Time: 5 minutes

Servings: 2

Nutrition: Calories 72, fats 6.3g, protein 0.7g, **carbs 4.5g**

Ingredients:

- ¾ c. Green beans
- 3 tsp. Minced garlic
- 2 tbsps. Rosemary
- ½ tsp. Salt
- 1 tbsp. Butter

Directions:

1. Warm-up an air fryer to 390°f.
2. Put the chopped green beans then brush with butter.
3. Sprinkle salt, minced garlic, and rosemary over then cook within 5 minutes.
4. Serve.

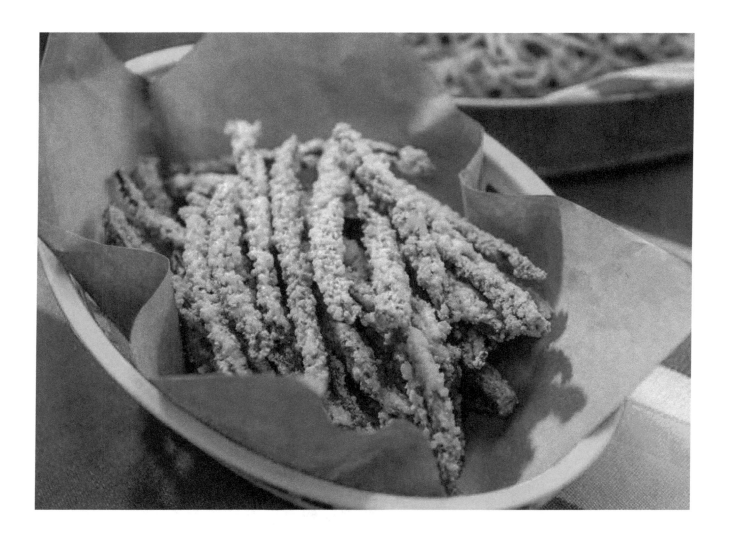

40. Low Carb Spinach & Cheddar

Preparation Time: 15 minutes

Cooking Time: 30 minutes

Servings: 8

Nutrition: Calories 365, fats 34.6g, protein 10.4g, **carbs 4.**

Ingredients:
- 3 c. Cream cheese
- 1½ c. Coconut flour
- 3 egg yolks
- 2 eggs
- ½ c. Cheddar cheese
- 2 c. Steamed spinach
- ¼ tsp. Salt
- ½ tsp. Pepper
- ¼ c. Onion

Directions:
1. Whisk cream cheese put egg yolks. Stir in coconut flour until becoming soft dough.
2. Put the dough on a flat surface then roll until thin. Cut the thin dough into 8 squares.
3. Beat the eggs, and then place it in a bowl. Put salt, pepper, and grated cheese.
4. Put chopped spinach and onion to the egg batter.
5. Put spinach filling on a square dough then fold until becoming an envelope. Glue with water.
6. Warm-up an air fryer to 425°f (218°c). Cook within 12 minutes.
7. Remove and serve!

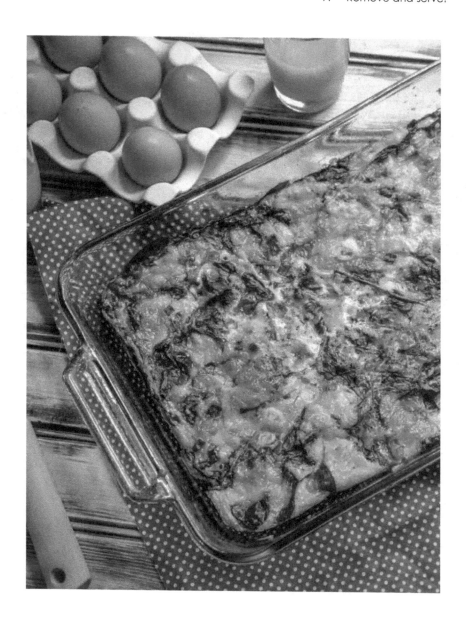

41. Almond Keto Cheese

Preparation Time: 10 minutes

Cooking Time: 15 minutes

Servings: 8

Nutrition: Calories: 365, fats 34.6g, protein 10.4g, **carbs 4.4g**

Ingredients:
- 2 c. Mushrooms
- 2 eggs
- ¾ c. Almond flour
- ½ c. Cheddar cheese
- 2 tbsps. Butter
- ½ tsp. Pepper
- ¼ tsp. Salt

Directions:
1. Processes chopped mushrooms in a food processor then add eggs, almond flour, and cheddar cheese.
2. Put salt and pepper then pour melted butter into the food processor. Transfer.
3. Warm-up an air fryer to 375°f (191°c).
4. Put the loaf pan on the air fryer's rack then cook within 15 minutes.
5. Slice and serve.

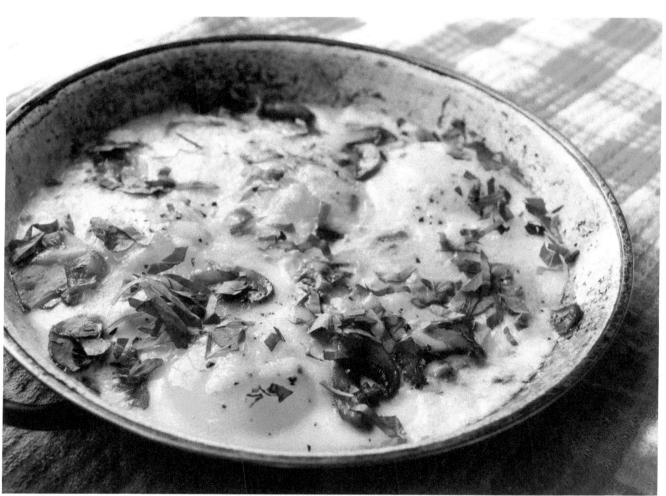

42. Mexican Low Carb Guacamole

Preparation Time: 10 minutes

Cooking Time: -

Servings: 4

Nutrition: Calories 16.5, fats 1.4g, protein 0.23g, **carbs: 0.5g**

Ingredients:

- Organic avocados pitted – 2
- Organic red onion – 1/3
- Organic jalapeño – 1
- Salt – ½ teaspoon
- Ground pepper – ½ teaspoon
- Tomato salsa – 2 tablespoons
- Lime juice – 1 tablespoon
- Organic cilantro – ½

Directions:

1. Slice the avocado flesh horizontally and vertically.
2. Mix in onion, jalapeno, and lime juice in a bowl.
3. Put salt and black pepper, add salsa and mix.
4. Fold in cilantro and serve.

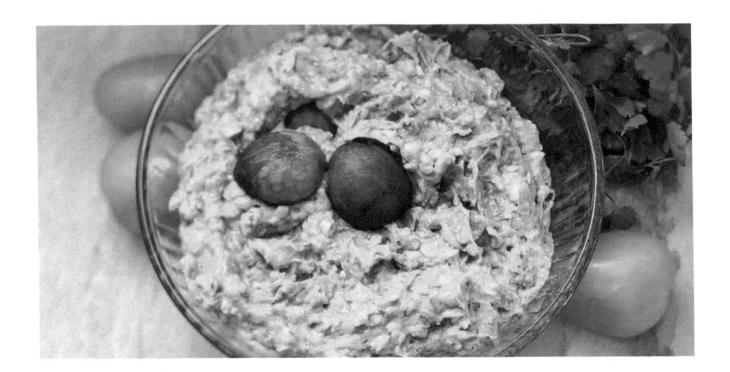

43. Raspberry Low Carb Mousse

Preparation Time: 5 minutes

Cooking Time: -

Servings: 2

Nutrition: Calories 254, Fats 9 g, **Carbs 1.2 g**, Protein 7.5 g

Ingredients:

- 2 cups heavy whipping cream
- 3 oz. fresh raspberries
- 2 oz. chopped pecans
- ½ lemon, zested
- ¼ tsp vanilla extract

Direction:

1. Beat cream in a bowl using a hand mixer until it forms peaks.
2. Stir in vanilla and lemon zest and mix well until incorporated.
3. Fold in nuts and berries and mix well.
4. Cover the mixture with plastic wrap and refrigerate for 3 hours.
5. Serve fresh.

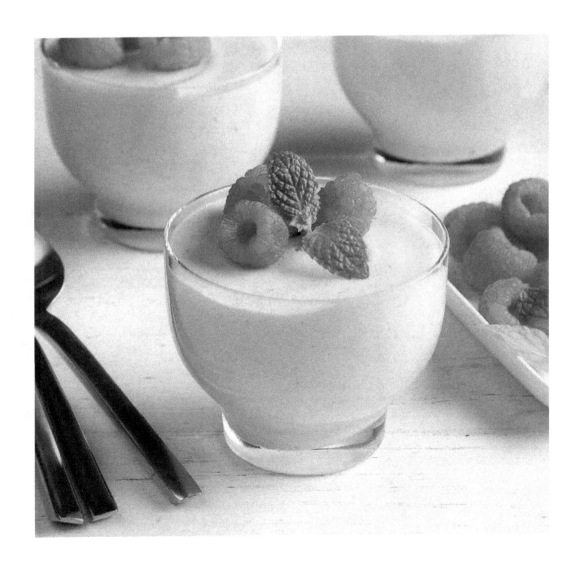

44. Keto Vegan Bites

Preparation Time: 10 minutes

Cooking Time: -

Servings: 3

Nutrition: 164 Calories, 16.3g Fats, **3g Carbs**, 2g Protein

Ingredients:

- 1 teaspoon Dijon mustard
- 1/2 cup cream cheese
- 1/4 cup mayonnaise
- 1 cucumber, cut into rounds
- 1 bell pepper, deveined and cut into 4 pieces lengthwise
- 1 teaspoon paprika

Direction:

1. Mix the Dijon mustard, cream cheese, and mayonnaise in a bowl; stir to combine.
2. Place the cucumber and bell peppers on a serving platter. Divide the cheese mixture between the vegetables.
3. Sprinkle paprika over the vegetable bites. Serve well chilled and enjoy!

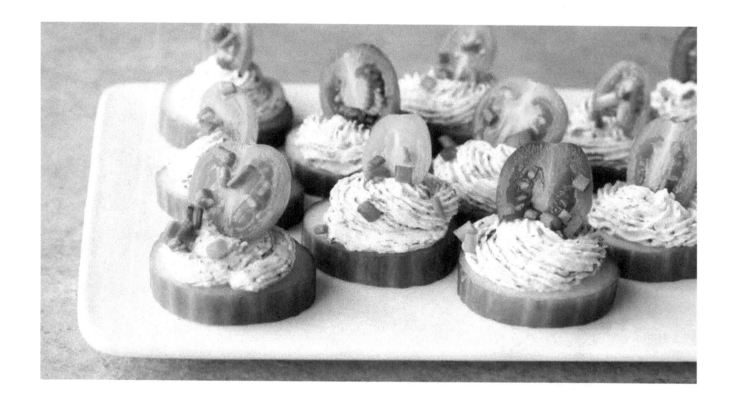

45. Ham & Cheesy Keto Balls

Preparation Time: 10 minutes

Cooking Time: -

Servings: 4

Nutrition: 76 Calories, 12.9g Fats, 2.3g Carbs, 12.8g Protein

Ingredients:

- 2 ounces goat cheese, crumbled
- 2 ounces feta cheese crumbled
- 3 ounces prosciutto, chopped
- 1 red bell pepper, deveined and finely chopped
- 2 tablespoons sesame seeds, toasted

Direction:

1. Thoroughly combine the cheese, prosciutto and pepper until everything is well incorporated. Shape the mixture into balls.

2. Arrange these keto balls on a platter and place them in the refrigerator until ready to serve.

3. Roll the keto balls in toasted sesame seeds before serving. Enjoy!!

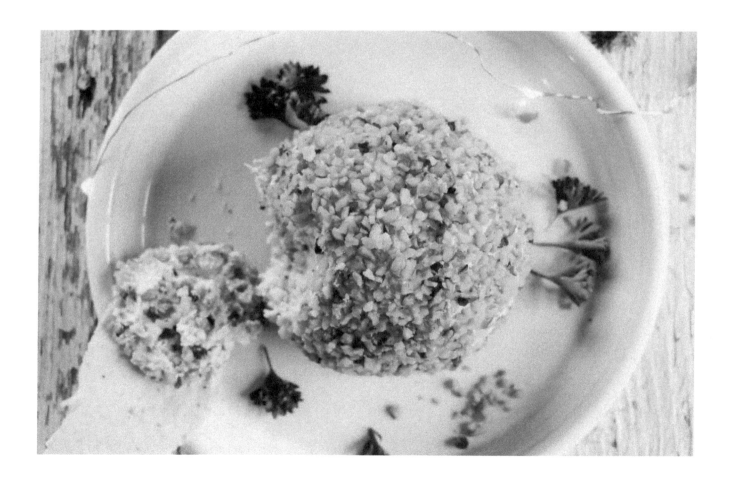

8. KETO DESSERT RECIPES

46. Low Carb Choco Brownies

Preparation Time: 30 minutes

Cooking Time: 20 minutes

Servings: 12

Nutrition: Calories 183.7, fats 16.6g, **carbs 4.9 g**, protein 1.4 g

Ingredients:

- 6 ounces coconut oil; melted
- 4 ounces cream cheese
- 5 tablespoons swerve
- 6 eggs
- 2 teaspoons vanilla
- 3 ounces of cocoa powder
- 1/2 teaspoon baking powder

Direction:

1. In a blender, mix eggs with coconut oil, cocoa powder, baking powder, vanilla, cream cheese, and swerve and stir using a mixer.
2. Pour this into a lined baking dish, introduce in the oven at 350 degrees f and bake for 20 minutes

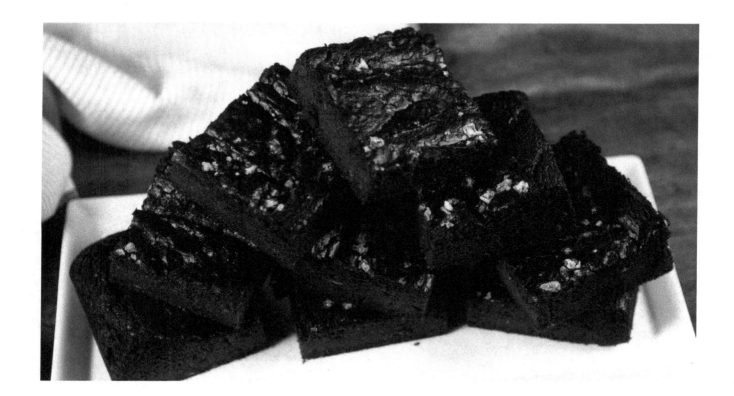

47. Cinnamon Muffin

Cooking Time: 12 minutes

Servings: 2

Nutrition: Calories 241, fats protein 7g, **carbs 3 g**

- 6 2/3 tbsp coconut flour
- ½ of egg
- 1 tbsp butter, unsalted, melted
- 1 1/3 tbsp whipping cream
- 1 tbsp almond milk, unsweetened

Others:
- 1 1/3 tbsp erythritol sweetener and more for topping
- ¼ tsp baking powder
- ¼ tsp ground cinnamon and more for topping
- ¼ tsp vanilla extract, unsweetened

1. Turn on the oven, then set it to 350 degrees f and let it preheat.
2. Meanwhile, take a medium bowl, place flour in it, add cinnamon, baking powder, and cinnamon and stir until combined.
3. Take a separate bowl, place the half egg in it, add butter, sour cream, milk, and vanilla and whisk until blended.
4. Whisk in flour mixture into incorporated and smooth batter comes together, divide the batter evenly between two silicon muffin cups and then sprinkle cinnamon and sweetener on top.
5. Bake the muffins for 10 to 12 minutes until firm, and then the top has turned golden brown and then serve and

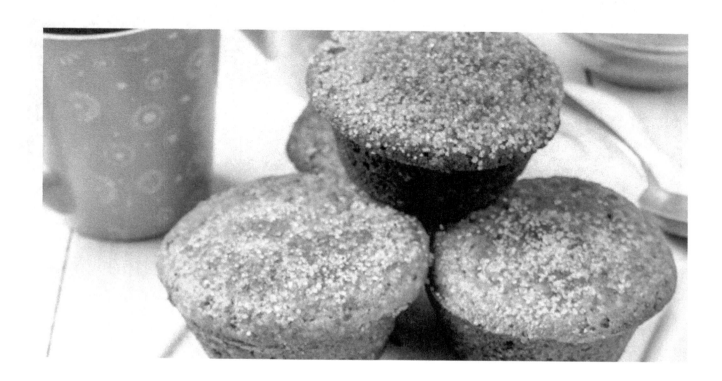

48. Almond & Berries Yogurt

Preparation Time: 5 minutes

Cooking Time: -

Servings: 2

Nutrition: Calories 165, fats 11.2g, protein 9.3g, **carbs 2.5 g**

Ingredients:
- 3 oz mixed berries
- 1 tbsp chopped almonds
- 1 tbsp chopped walnuts
- 4 oz yogurt

Directions:
1. Divide yogurt between two bowls, top with berries, and then sprinkle with almonds and walnuts.
2. Serve and enjoy!

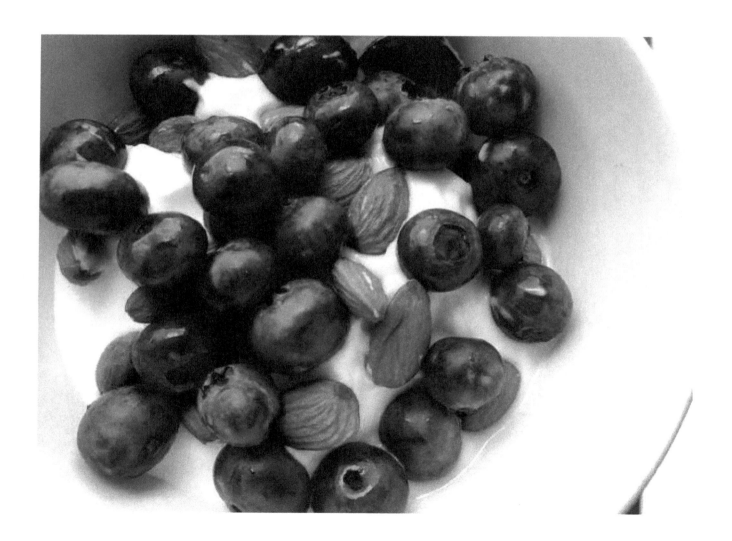

49. Keto Cupcakes

Preparation Time: 5 minutes

Cooking Time: 15 minutes

Servings: 9

Nutrition: 163 Calories, 17g Fats, **1.5g Carbs**, 2.3g Protein

Ingredients:

- 6 eggs, beaten
- 1/2 cup coconut oil, melted
- 3 tablespoons granulated Swerve
- 2 tablespoons flaxseed meal
- 1/3 cup coconut flour
- 1 teaspoon baking powder
- A pinch of salt
- A pinch of freshly grated nutmeg
- 1 teaspoon lemon zest
- 1 teaspoon coconut extract

Directions:

1. Start by preheating your oven to 360 degrees F. Coat a muffin pan with cupcake liners.
2. Beat the eggs with the coconut oil and granulated Swerve until frothy.
3. In another mixing bowl, thoroughly combine the remaining ingredients.
4. Stir this dry mixture into the wet mixture; mix again to combine.
5. Spoon the batter into the prepared muffin pan.
6. Bake for 13 to 15 minutes, or until a tester comes out dry and clean.
7. To serve, sprinkle with some extra granulated Swerve if desired.

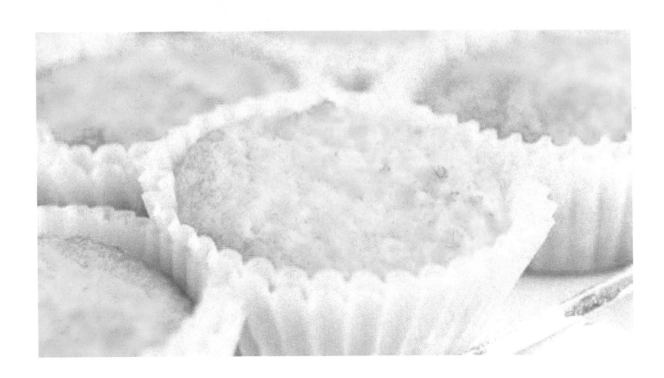

50. *Tahini Bars*

Preparation Time: 5 minutes

Cooking Time: 1 minute + 40 minutes chilling time

Servings: 10

Nutrition: 176 Calories, 18.3g Fats, **3.2g Carbs**, 1.8g Protein

Ingredients:

- 1/2 stick butter
- 2 tablespoons tahini (sesame paste)
- 1/2 cup almond butter
- 1 teaspoon Stevia
- 2 ounces baker's chocolate, sugar-free
- A pinch of salt
- A pinch of grated nutmeg
- 1/2 teaspoon cinnamon powder

Directions:

1. Microwave the butter for 30 to 35 seconds. Fold in the tahini, almond butter, Stevia, and chocolate.

2. Sprinkle with salt, nutmeg, and cinnamon; whisk to combine well. Scrape the mixture into a parchment-lined baking tray.

3. Transfer to the freezer for 40 minutes. Cut into bars and enjoy!

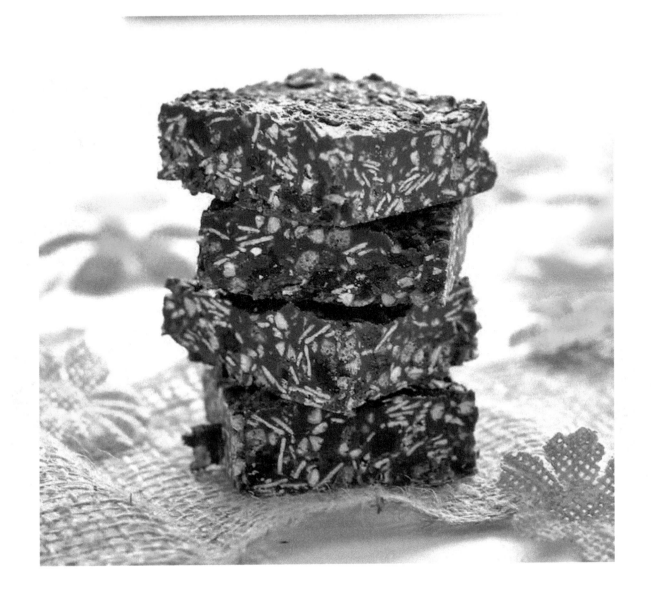

51. Choco Cube

Preparation Time: 55 minutes

Cooking Time: 1 minute

Servings: 10

Nutrition: 234 Calories, 25.1g Fats, **3.6g Carbs**, 1.7g Protein

Ingredients:
- 1/2 cup coconut flour
- 1/2 cup almond meal
- 1 cup almond butter
- 1/4 cup erythritol
- 2 tablespoons coconut oil
- 1/2 cup sugar-free bakers' chocolate, chopped into small chunks

Directions:
1. Mix the coconut flour, almond meal, butter, and erythritol until smooth.
2. Press the mixture into a parchment-lined square pan. Place in your freezer for 30 minutes.
3. Meanwhile, microwave the coconut oil and bakers' chocolate for 40 seconds.
4. Pour the glaze over the cake and transfer to your freezer until the chocolate is set or about 20 minutes.
5. Cut into cube and enjoy!

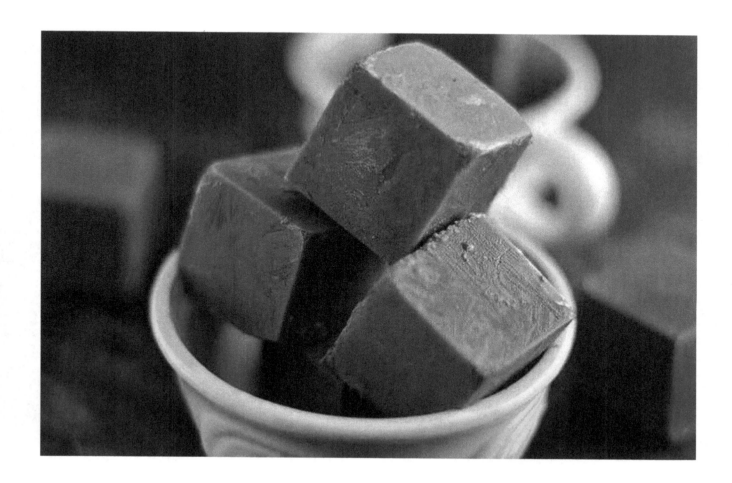

52. Jack Sparrow Cookies

Preparation Time: 10 minutes

Cooking Time: 3 hours chilling time

Servings: 12

Nutrition: 400 Calories, 40g Fats, **4.9g Carbs,** 5.4g Protein

Ingredients:
- 1/2 cup coconut butter
- 1/2 stick butter
- 1/2 cup almond butter
- 1/2 cup confectioners' Swerve
- 1 teaspoon rum extract
- 2 cups almond meal
- 2 cups pork rinds, crushed
- 1/2 cup chocolate chips, sugar-free

Directions:
1. Microwave the coconut butter, butter, and almond butter until melted.
2. Add in the Swerve and rum extract. After that, add in the almond meal, pork rinds, and chocolate chips.
3. Form balls with a cookie scoop and then, shape the mixture into 12 cookies.
4. Refrigerate at least 3 hours so they can firm up completely. Enjoy!

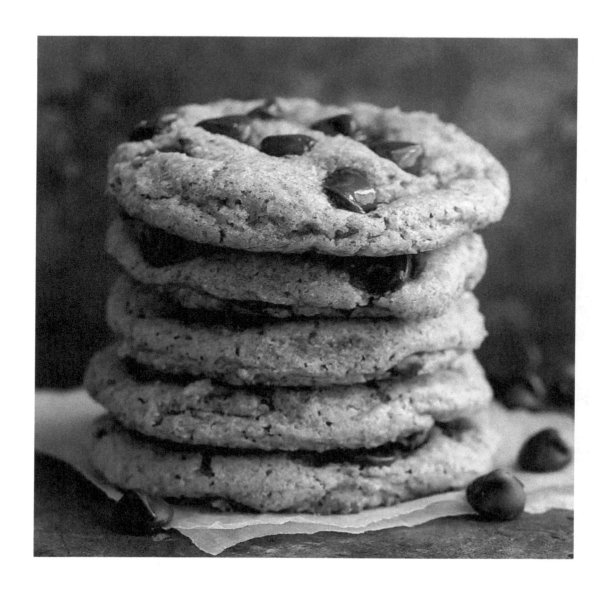

53. Keto Pudding

Preparation Time: 5 minutes

Cooking Time: 20 minutes

Servings: 4

Nutrition: 214 Calories, 21g Fats, **1.7g Carbs**, 5g Protein

Ingredients:

- 2 eggs
- A pinch of flaky salt
- 2 egg yolks
- 1 vanilla bean
- 4 tablespoons granulated Swerve
- 1 ½ cups heavy whipping cream
- 1/4 teaspoon ground cloves
- 1/4 teaspoon ground cinnamon

Directions:

1. Carefully separate the egg whites from the yolks. Whip the egg whites just until a bit foamy. Add in a pinch of salt and beat the eggs until soft peaks have formed. Set aside.

2. In a sauté pan, place the egg yolks, vanilla, Swerve and cream. Let it simmer over moderate flame until thickened and thoroughly heated, about 20 minutes.

3. Add in the ground cloves and cinnamon; mix again to combine well.

4. Remove from the heat and fold in the reserved egg whites; gently stir to combine and let it cool to room temperature.

5. Place in your refrigerator until ready to use.

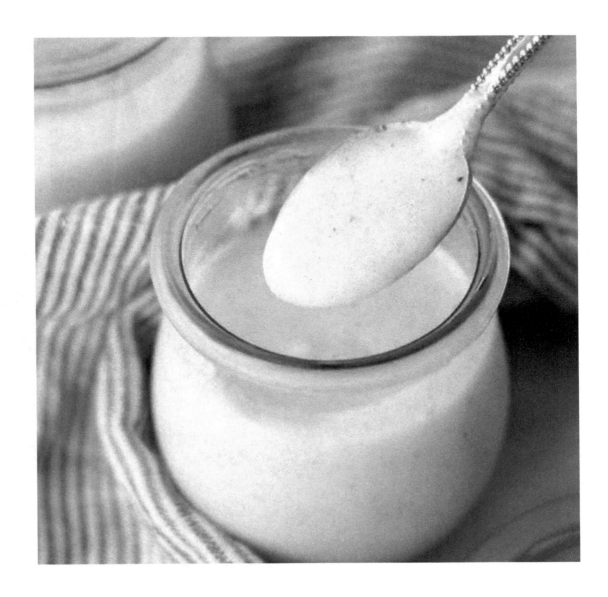

54. Vitamin keto Cheesecake

Preparation Time: 10 minutes

Cooking Time: 5 minutes

Servings: 12

Nutrition: 150 Calories, 15.4g Fats, **2.1g Carbs,** 1.2g Protein

Ingredients:
- 1 tablespoon Swerve
- 1 cup almond flour
- 1 stick butter, room temperature
- 1/2 cup unsweetened coconut, shredded

Filling:
- 1 teaspoon powdered gelatin
- 2 tablespoons Swerve
- 17 ounces mascarpone cream
- 2 tablespoon orange juice

Directions:
1. Thoroughly combine all the ingredients for the crust; press the crust mixture into a lightly greased baking dish.
2. Let it stand in your refrigerator.
3. Then, mix 1 cup of boiling water and gelatin until all dissolved. Pour in 1 cup of cold water.
4. Add Swerve, mascarpone cheese, and orange juice; blend until smooth and uniform. Pour the filling onto the prepared crust. Enjoy!

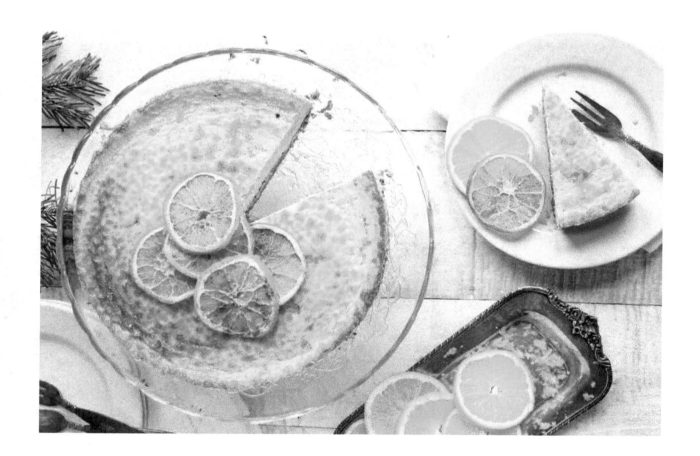

55. Halloween Keto Cup

Preparation Time: 10 minutes

Cooking Time: 12 minutes

Servings: 2

Nutrition: Calories 261, fats 23g, protein 7g, **carbs 2 g**

Ingredients:

- 4 tbsp almond flour
- 1 1/3 tbsp coconut flour
- 2 tbsp pumpkin puree
- 2 2/3 tbsp cream cheese, softened
- ½ of egg
- 2/3 tbsp butter, unsalted
- ¼ tsp pumpkin spice
- 2/3 tsp baking powder
- 2 tbsp erythritol sweetener

Directions:

1. Turn on the oven, then set it to 350 degrees f and let it preheat.
2. Take a medium bowl, place butter and 1 ½ tbsp sweetener in it, and then beat until fluffy.
3. Beat in egg and then beat in pumpkin puree until well combined.
4. Take a medium bowl, place flours in it, stir in pumpkin spice, baking powder until mixed, stir this mixture into the butter mixture and then distribute the mixture into two silicone muffin cups.
5. Take a medium bowl, place cream cheese in it, and stir in remaining sweetener until well combined.
6. Divide the cream cheese mixture into the silicone muffin cups, swirl the batter and cream cheese mixture by using a toothpick and then bake for 10 to 12 minutes until muffins have turned firm.
7. Serve and enjoy!

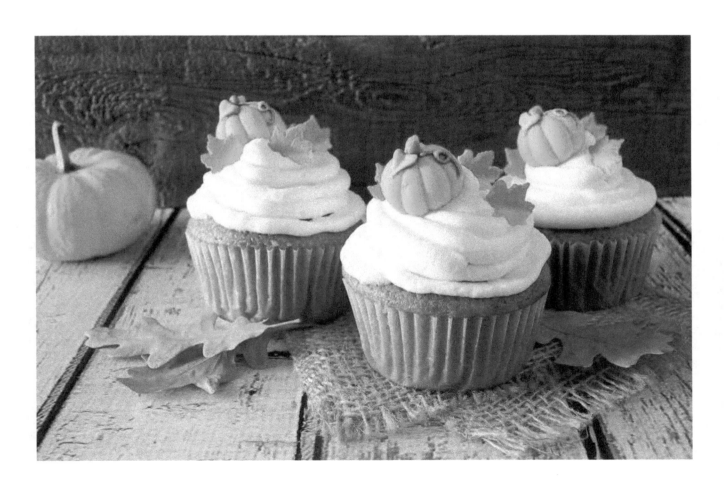

9 781801 645324